Conception and Family Planning - New Aspects

Edited by Panagiotis Tsikouras,
Nikolaos Nikolettos, Werner Rath
and Friedrich Von Tempelhoff

Published in London, United Kingdom

Conception and Family Planning - New Aspects
http://dx.doi.org/10.5772/intechopen.110909
Edited by Panagiotis Tsikouras, Nikolaos Nikolettos, Werner Rath and Friedrich Von Tempelhoff

Contributors
Abdulai Abubakari, Abraham Alano, Alexios Alexiou, Alfred A. Shihata, Anastasia Bothou, Anna Maria Paoletti, Anna Melis, Arabatzis John, Athanasia Hatzilazarou, Athanasia Kassapi, Birgit Linderoth, Bruno Piras, Dimitios Kyriakou, Elena Giancane, Ethimios Oikonomou, Georgios Iatrakis, Gian Benedetto Melis, Giulia Melis, Hanny-Sherry Ayittey, Jude Anim, Konstantnos Nikolettos, Leena Uppal, Lori Hanson, Manuela Neri, Maria Francesca Marotto, Maria Georganta, Mathoka Khaile, Metella Dei, Monica Pilloni, Naana Boadiwaa Asante, Natalia Sachnova, Nikolaos Nikolettos, Panagiotis Tsikouras, Pierina Zedda, Priyanka Rani Garg, Rahma Salifu, Raida Koray, Richard Grossman, Steven A. Brody, Sunil Mehra, Theopi Nalbanti, Valeria Taccori, Valerio Vallerino, Vincenzina Bruni, Virginia Melis

First published in London, United Kingdom, 2024 by IntechOpen
IntechOpen is the global imprint of INTECHOPEN LIMITED, registered in England and Wales, registration number: 11086078, 167-169 Great Portland Street, London, W1W 5PF, United Kingdom

British Library Cataloguing-in-Publication Data
A catalogue record for this book is available from the British Library

Additional hard and PDF copies can be obtained from orders@intechopen.com

Conception and Family Planning - New Aspects
Edited by Panagiotis Tsikouras, Nikolaos Nikolettos, Werner Rath and Friedrich Von Tempelhoff
p. cm.

This title is part of the Obstetrics and Gynecology Book Series, Volume 2
Topic: Reproductive and Gynecologic Health
Series Editor: Zouhair O. Amarin
Topic Editor: Courtney Marsh

Print ISBN 978-1-83768-147-1
Online ISBN 978-1-83768-148-8
eBook (PDF) ISBN 978-1-83768-208-9
ISSN 3049-706X

An electronic version of this book is freely available, thanks to the partial funding support of libraries working with Knowledge Unlatched. KU is a collaborative initiative designed to make high quality books Open Access for the public good. More information about the initiative and links to the Open Access version can be found at www.knowledgeunlatched.org

IntechOpen Book Series

Obstetrics and Gynecology

Volume 2

Aims and Scope of the Series

Obstetrics and Gynecology field typically covers several subspecialties that include maternal-fetal medicine, gynecologic oncology, reproductive endocrinology and subfertility, urogynecology and female pelvic reconstructive surgery, critical care medicine, complex family planning, pediatric and adolescent gynecology, menopausal and geriatric gynecology, and minimally invasive gynecologic surgery.
Apart from being diverse, obstetrics and gynecology is a challenging and demanding specialty. It combines medical and surgical skills.
The sequence of books in this series will have certain characteristics in common that will be recognized as part of the same informative multi-volume book programme.

Meet the Series Editor

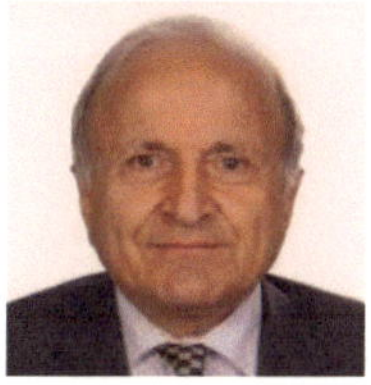

Zouhair Amarin is a Professor of Obstetrics and Gynaecology at the Jordan University of Science and Technology. He was previously a lecturer at the University of Glasgow, Scotland, a senior lecturer at the University of Nottingham, England, and the dean of the Faculty of Medicine at Mutah University, Jordan. Professor Amarin is a fellow of the Royal College of Obstetricians and Gynaecologists, and the Faculty of Public Health, London. He holds master's degrees in medical science and medical education. He is a pioneer in IVF and was the first in the world to develop microsurgical epididymis sperm aspiration for clinical use. He also discovered a surgical procedure for critical ovarian hyperstimulation syndrome. Professor Amarin has edited books, authored book chapters, and published more than 130 papers. He is the recipient of eight awards.

Meet the Volume Editors

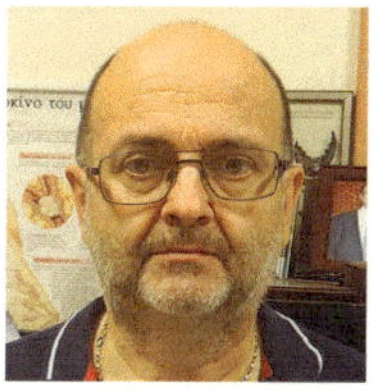

Panagiotis Tsikouras is a specialist professor in obstetrics and gynecology, perinatal medicine, and contraception at the School of Medicine, Democritus University of Thrace, Greece. He is also head of the Family Planning Centre and Gynecological Cytology Laboratory at the same university. Dr. Tsikouras is a fellow of the International Academy of Clinical and Applied Thrombosis/Hemostasis. His scientific activities focus on pediatric and adolescent medicine, gynecological oncology, and high-risk pregnancies. He is a reviewer for several international journals and has numerous scientific publications to his credit, including papers and book chapters. He has also contributed to international and national guidelines on coagulation and thrombosis in obstetrics and gynecology.

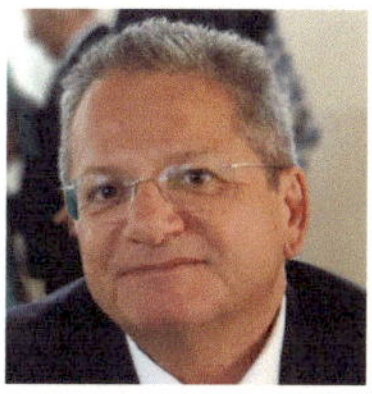

Prof. Nikolettos Nikos is a Professor of Obstetrics and Gynecology and Assisted Reproduction at the Democritus University of Thrace, Greece. He has training in gynecological endocrinology, human reproduction, and in vitro fertilization. From 2007 to 2011, he was the director of the In Vitro Fertilization Unit, University Regional General Hospital of Alexandroupolis, Greece. From 2012 to 2018, he was the director of the Laboratory of Reproductive Physiology-Artificial Fertilization. In 2019, he took over the management of the University Obstetrics-Gynecology Clinic of the Medical Department at the same university. His scientific work includes more than 100 publications in international journals and numerous invited lectures at international and Greek conferences.

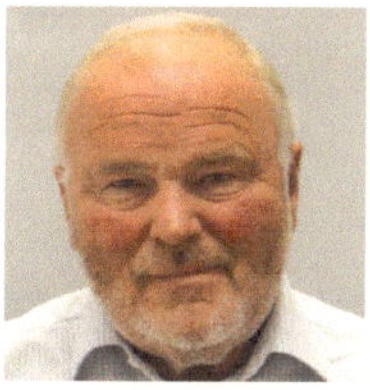

Prof. Dr. h. c. Werner Rath is a specialist professor in obstetrics and gynecology, gynecologic oncology, perinatal medicine, and hemostaseology. He was chief of the Department of Gynecology and Obstetrics, University Hospital Aachen, Germany. He is a Professor of Gynecology and Obstetrics in the Faculty of Medicine, University Kiel, Germany. He is an honorary doctor at the University of Alexandroupolis, Greece. Dr. Rath is the recipient of several awards, including the Staude-Pfannenstiel Award of the North Germany Society of Gynecology and Obstetrics, Maternité Award from the German Society of Perinatal Medicine, and the Berlin Harald-Bräutigam Award. He is a reviewer for numerous national and international journals and was editor-in-chief of the Journal Geburtshilfe and Frauenheilkunde and Zeitschrift für Geburtshilfe Und Neonatologie (Thieme Publisher) for many years.

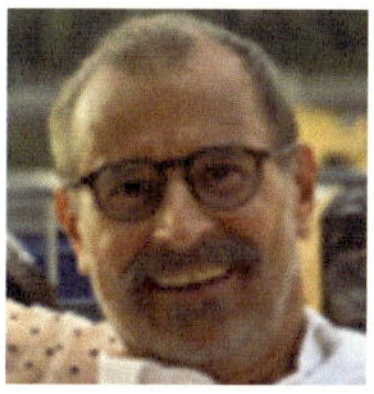

Prof. Dr. George Friedrich von Tempelhoff, FCATH, is a specialist professor in obstetrics and gynecology, gynecologic oncology, perinatal medicine, and hemostaseology. He is chief of the Department of Gynecology and Obstetrics, St. Vinzensius Hospital, Hanau Germany, and head of the Institute for Thrombosis and Coagulation Disorders in Gynecology and Obstetrics, Germany. He completed his medical education at Justus-Liebig University, Germany, and became a Consultant of Obstetrics and Gynecology in 1996. He received his doctorate in medicine in 1993 and completed his habilitation at the Johannes-Gutenberg University Mainz, Germany in 2007. He was appointed extracurricular professor at the Julius-Maximilians-Universität Würzburg, Germany in 2015. He is a fellow of the International Academy of Clinical and Applied Thrombosis/Hemostasis. His scientific focus is on hemostaseological and hemorheological disorders in women with miscarriages, preeclampsia, and thrombosis. Dr. Tempelhoff is a reviewer for numerous journals, author of several publications and book chapters, and a contributor to international and national guidelines on coagulation and thrombosis in gynecology.

Contents

Preface

The purpose of contraception is to prevent an egg from being fertilized by sperm or to prevent the implantation of a fertilized egg in the uterus. There are many methods of contraception. The ideal method of contraception will prevent pregnancy and protect against sexually transmitted diseases. It is essential to understand and approach each method according to the person's sexual needs. Unfortunately, many people of reproductive age do not have access to contraceptive counseling and services. In developing countries, most pregnancies occur in young and teenage women, unexpectedly and undesirably. Approximately 50% of these pregnancies are artificially terminated under unsafe conditions.

Contraception, especially hormonal contraception, has protective characteristics for those who take it, especially in young adolescence. Contraception was practiced for decades on an empirical basis, but the discovery of the contraceptive pill brought about a real revolution in this field. By using scientific techniques, we managed to prevent ovulation, which is the cornerstone of reproduction. Since the outbreak of AIDS, the usage of birth control pills has decreased because they do not offer any protection against sexually transmitted diseases. On the contrary, barrier contraception that offers protection from STDs prevents direct contact. The contraceptive pill continues to be a unique scientific achievement, which if combined with intrauterine devices creates a protective shield against unwanted pregnancy. The clinical implementation of oral contraception dates back to the 1960s, but its history goes back to the beginning of the 20th century when experimental data showed that the ovaries were organs with hormonal activity. Adolescence is a period in which many physical, emotional, and psychological changes occur in a relatively short time. In this context, one's sexuality, especially in young girls, is developed, with young women particularly vulnerable to possible unwanted pregnancies and STDs. The ever-decreasing age of onset of sexual relations that has been observed worldwide in recent years urges the need for proper sex education and informing teenagers about their contraceptive options. Undoubtedly, accessing information is extremely easy, but there are still many misunderstandings about the methods of contraception today.

The factors that determine whether pregnancy will take place include the fertility of both partners, the year of having intercourse in relation to the time of ovulation, the method of contraception used, and the endogenous efficiency as well as the correct usage of the method. It is impossible to approximate the effectiveness of a contraceptive method isolated from the other factors. Besides effectiveness, contraceptive methods are evaluated by their side effects, ease of implementation, reversibility, and acceptance by the population. The best way to determine the effectiveness of a contraceptive method is by long-term evaluation of a group of sexually active women who use the specific method for a particular period and observing how often pregnancy occurs. The failure rate of each contraceptive method expressed as pregnancies per 100 women per year, is determined by calculating the Pearl Index specific to each method. This involves dividing the number of pregnancies by the total number of months in the observed period for the pairs and then multiplying the resulting quotient by 1200. A method is considered effective when the number of unwanted pregnancies is less than 2 in 100 women who use the method for a year, moderately effective when the rate of unintended pregnancies is up to 10%, and less effective when the rate of unwanted pregnancies is more than 10%. The efficiency of a method can thus be expressed with two values. The one value results from the set of pairs in which the contraceptive method is used as usual. Therefore, a particular method may be effective for one couple, but not for others. That is, it is a kind of average price effectiveness. The other value refers to the percentage of unwanted pregnancies when the method is used optimally, that is, when used correctly and consistently.

Currently, the World Health Organization (WHO) recommends a 24-month postpartum interval for a subsequent pregnancy. It is estimated that effective family planning globally could prevent 1 in 10 deaths among fetuses by helping women to give birth at least 2 years later because a short period of less than 12 months between pregnancies increases the risk of complications such as low birth weight, premature birth, stillbirth, and neonatal death. Defining contraceptive failure is not easy, as it depends on the population studied. Studies in a young population will suggest a higher failure rate than in an older age group, as fertility is higher in younger people. Consequently, caution is required when interpreting the relevant numbers. "Method failure" includes the inherent risk of failure provided the method is used properly. Percentages are measured in units per 100 women years to the number of women who would become pregnant if 100 of them used this method of contraception for one year. User failure is the failure rate when the method is not used correctly (missed tablets, delayed injections, drug interactions).

With proper guidance from family planning centers, if used consistently and correctly, hormonal contraception (combined hormonal methods, progestogen-only pills, injectables, implants, and intrauterine devices) and non-hormonal methods (copper intrauterine devices [Cu-IUD], sterilization in males and females) are more than 99% effective in preventing pregnancy.

Panagiotis Tsikouras and Nikolaos Nikolettos
Professor,
Department of Obstetrics and Gynecology,
Democritus University of Thrace,
Alexandroupolis, Greece

Werner Rath
Professor,
Gynecology and Obstetrics in the Faculty of Medicine,
University of Kiel,
Kiel, Germany

Friedrich Von Tempelhoff
Professor,
Gynecology and Obstetrics,
St. Vinzenz Teaching Hospital,
Hanau, Germany

Section 1

Contraception in Adolescents

Chapter 1

Adolescents' Access to Contraception in Lesotho: A Gender and Social Inclusion Perspective

Mathoka Khaile

Abstract

Adolescents' access to contraception is a serious global and regional concern as a public health component. Therefore, this chapter analyses adolescents' access to contraception, using gender and social inclusion lens, where the access to contraception services and information is explored. Thus, legislative and administrative measures as well as practices focusing on access to contraception are analysed in this chapter, using desk review and content analysis from the gender and social inclusion perspective. The results reveal that Lesotho is a state party to treaties that obligate states to ensure access to contraception for adolescents from the gender and social inclusion perspective, and this has also been implicated in the Constitution of Lesotho. However, other laws do not provide for gender- and social-inclusive access to contraception for adolescents. Administratively, the National Family Planning Guidelines for Health Service Providers of 2017 and National Strategic Development Plan II are the only strategies that are gender-responsive and use social inclusion lens to facilitate access to contraception for adolescents. Other policies are gender-blind and silent about adolescents and access to contraception. Lastly, statistics show that many adolescents do not have access to contraception, and gender- and social-inclusion issues are not taken into consideration.

Keywords: adolescents, access, contraception, gender, social inclusion

1. Introduction

Contraception is one of the most significant determinants of fertility in developing countries [1]. The World Health Organisation emphasises that there is no method of contraception contraindicated on the basis of age alone [2]. Thus, this statement extends to adolescents who have the right to sexual and reproductive health services, including contraceptive care and counselling [3]. However, adolescents' access to contraception is a serious global and regional concern as a public health component [4]. Hence, Cook and Dickens argue that national healthcare services fail to respond to sexual and reproductive health needs of adolescents [5]. In addition, adolescents of Lesotho have a challenge of accessing contraception at the health facilities [6], thereby increasing the vulnerability of adolescents to pregnancy and sexually transmitted infections [7]. Adolescence is a challenging stage for young people who rely on 'their families, peers, schools and health service providers for affirmation, advice, information and the skills to navigate the sometimes difficult transition to adulthood' [8]. For instance, statistics reveal that adolescents engage in sexual debut at a progressively younger age [9, 10], and this practice is linked to an increase in teenage pregnancy and sexually transmitted infections (see [7], p. 136). 50% of teenage pregnancies are unintended and result from low contraceptive usage [11].

Besides challenges faced by adolescents globally and regionally, the Government of Lesotho has made some strides to provide contraception to adolescents with the aim of promoting sexual and reproductive health and rights in the country. In this endeavour, the government is supported by development partners, international nongovernmental organisations and the civil society. Nevertheless, it is not clear if the access to contraception for adolescents has gender and social integration, even though it is expected that access to contraception is experienced differently by different groups of adolescents in the society in terms of gender, disability, geographic location and education. It has been noted that adolescents are a heterogeneous group. Therefore, it is significant to examine how adolescent girls and boys, as well as other socially excluded adolescents, have access to contraception in Lesotho. Thus, legislative and administrative measures as well as practices focusing on access to contraception shall be discussed in this chapter, using desk review and content analysis from the gender- and social-inclusion perspective.

2. International human rights law and adolescents' access to contraception

Articles 2, 11 and 18 of the Vienna Convention on the Law of Treaties provide that once a state party accedes to an international or regional treaty, it is bound by the treaty and has to refrain from acts that would impede the achievement of the treaty's objectives and purpose [12]. Therefore, human rights treaties, of which Lesotho has ratified or acceded to, are binding, and they are analysed in relation to the adolescents' access to contraception through gender- and social-inclusion lens. The following human rights treaties are ratified by Lesotho and are analysed in this section: International Covenant on Economic, Social and Cultural Rights (ICESCR), Convention on the Elimination of All Forms of Discrimination against Women (CEDAW), Convention on the Rights of the Child (CRC), Convention on the Rights of Persons with Disabilities (CRPD), African Charter on Human and Peoples' Rights (Banjul Charter) and Protocol to the African Charter on Human and Peoples' Rights on the Rights of Women in Africa (Maputo Protocol).

2.1 International covenant on economic, social and cultural rights

Article 12 of this covenant enjoins state parties to have the provision for the reduction of the stillbirth rate and infant mortality and for the healthy development of the child. In addition, according the General Comment 14 of the Committee on Economic, Social and Cultural Rights, access to sexual and reproductive health services should not be hindered by practices based on conscience. That is, provision of sexual and reproductive health services should not be hampered by conscientious objection. Although this article is not specific about adolescents' access to contraception as one of the sexual and reproductive services, it is relevant to adolescents' access to contraception because if they do not have access to contraception for controlling their fertility or reproduction, some adolescents are prone to having unhealthy child development due to not having been developed enough to take care of babies. Furthermore, when the adolescents do not have access to contraception, they are susceptible to having stillbirths and infant mortalities, as contraception is effective for preventing pregnancy and reducing its adverse effects among both adolescents and babies [13].

It is noted from the provisions of the ICESCR, especially article 12, that it does not have a gender- or social-inclusion lens for adolescents' access to contraception. It is gender-blind and does not integrate social-exclusion considerations related to access to contraception for adolescents in Lesotho. Therefore, the state is not bound by the treaty to ensure that different categories of adolescents in different geographic locations of Lesotho have equal access to contraception, thereby necessitating strengthening sexual and reproductive health for Basotho adolescents, especially access to contraception in order to prevent unintended pregnancies that may result in maternal death due to unsafe abortion. 'Unsafe abortions continue to contribute to high maternal death numbers in the SADC region' [14]. According to the United Nations Population Fund, governments are obliged to take affirmative actions that ensure adolescents' access to contraception in both law and practice, applying a human rights-based approach [15]. The UNFPA assertion implicates that the international and domestic laws need to make provisions for access to contraception for the adolescents, although the ICESCR is silent on this issue.

Nevertheless, the General Comment 14 of the Committee on Economic, Social and Cultural Rights (CESCR) expounds that access to contraception should not be impeded by practices based on conscience; thus, the International Covenant on Economic, Social and Cultural Rights is against a social norm of regarding contraception as a taboo for adolescents, thereby deterring adolescents' access to contraception. Thus, there is a need to adopt social norms approaches that will be used to challenge conscientious objection in relation to providing adolescents with contraception because of age. In accordance with social norms approaches, the misalignment between people's behaviours, attitudes and existing social norms should be harnessed in order to effect change [16]. Strategies could include changing gender norms and attitudes among an influential group [17]. Accordingly, there should be strategies geared towards changing gender norms and attitudes of policymakers as an influential group in relation to access to contraception by adolescents. Parents also need to be targeted as they have influence on adolescents, thereby controlling their access to contraception. Inversely, active participation of parents in ensuring access of contraception to adolescents will result in making supportive parents to adolescents' access to contraception. Adolescents are reluctant to seek sexual and reproductive health services because of systematic and legal barriers; adolescents also do not want their parents to find out that they are sexually active [18].

2.2 Convention on the elimination of all forms of discrimination against women

Article 12 Convention on the Elimination of All Forms of Discrimination against Women (CEDAW) provides that states parties should ensure equal access of men and women to health-care services related to family planning. Moreover, article 16 obligates states to ensure that women have a right to decide on the number of children to have and how to space them, and the CEDAW Committee General Recommendation

24 on article 12 states that women should not be impeded by states to pursue their health goals. A commitment to the two articles implicates that Lesotho is expected to avail equal access to sexual and reproductive health services, which include access to contraception, thereby including respecting other fundamental human rights. Cook asserts that the right to liberty and security of a person is violated when his/her fertility is denied by the state [19]. Therefore, Lesotho provides for access to contraception for adolescent girls concomitantly with CEDAW, even though it has been noted that the convention regards adolescent girls as a homogeneous group. Access to information about contraception and contraceptive services is determined by different factors such as literacy, age geographic location, disability and social norms.

Furthermore, the CEDAW Committee raised a concern about Basotho women's limited access to quality sexual and reproductive services in rural and remote areas [20]. As a result, the committee urges the state to ensure that women in rural areas and remote areas do not have barriers to access to family planning information and services and to promote education on sexual and reproductive health targeting adolescent girls and boys. Sochacki argues that the CEDAW Committee should do more to pressurise states parties to increase access to contraception as many international treaty-monitoring bodies have not fully exercised their powers to ensure that member states comply with ensuring access to contraception. It is against this backdrop that it has been discovered that although Lesotho has ratified CEDAW, thereby necessitating access to contraception by adolescent girls, there is no compliance to international law. Adolescent girls do not have access to contraception. Therefore, the CEDAW Committee needs to devise monitoring tools that will ensure that Lesotho ensures access to contraception for adolescents, using a gender- and social-inclusion lens in order to prevent maternal mortality and morbidity linked to adolescence. Culwell et al. state that states must provide enough health care to prevent maternal mortality and morbidity, as well as reduce unwanted pregnancies and unsafe abortions [21], as Maziwisa argues that the right to contraception is intricately linked to the right to life [see 18].

2.3 Convention on the rights of the child

Article 24 of the Convention on the Rights of the Child (CRC) obligates states parties to take effective and relevant measures to abolish traditional practices that are prejudicial to the health of children. Traditional practices which are detrimental to the health of children include teenage pregnancy or the practice of young mothers (young mothers are female adolescents who have babies), and the aforesaid practices affect both adolescent girls and boys, adolescents living in the urban or rural areas, literate or illiterate, and adolescents without or with disabilities. Cook asserts that article 9(1) of the International Covenant on Civil and Political Rights (ICCPR) read with article 19 of the CRC shows that lack of access to contraception-related information, education and services violates adolescent girls' rights to liberty and security of the person (see [19]). Therefore, impeding access to information and education about contraception by the adolescents is a violation of fundamental human rights.

Failure to ensure access to sexual and reproductive health and rights (SRHR) education results in increased risk of early pregnancies that may result in complications such as foetus loss, infant mortality and vesicovaginal fistulas for adolescent girls (see [19]). That is why Durojaye argues that there is a strong existing correlation between adolescent girls' literacy and sexual and reproductive health and rights [22]. 'Literacy facilitates access to SRHR information and can help reduce early pregnancies, STIs,

HIV, and early marriage, especially in the rural areas where adolescent-friendly services are not easily accessible' (see [18]). Therefore, states must facilitate education on the correct use and effects of contraceptives to enable adolescent girls to protect themselves when they begin exploring their sexuality (see [18]). Nevertheless, more focus on the raised arguments is based on adolescent girls as a homogenous group, not unpacking all groups of adolescents.

The Committee on the Rights of the Child General Comment No.20 states that all adolescents need access to confidential, adolescent-responsive and non-discriminatory sexual and reproductive health services that include contraception, because access to high-quality child-friendly sexual and reproductive health services could transform the situation [23]. In addition, General Comment No.4 emphasises that states should reduce maternal morbidity and mortality in adolescent girls. This implies that the practice of deterring adolescents from having access to contraception as a social-exclusion practice is a prejudice against adolescents which may negatively affect their health. In addition, article 3(1) of the CRC enjoins states parties to take all actions concerning children, prioritising the best interests of the child. Similarly, in cases where the child's views and/or interests are distinct from those of parents, the best-interests test can be used to legitimately respect the child's right to receive sexual and reproductive health services, including counselling and treatment, and override parental consent. Thus, failure to facilitate access to contraception by adolescents does not prioritise the principle of the best interest of the child because when adolescents prioritise not to bear children, yet there are no contraceptive services that help them prevent pregnancy; they are more prone to unintended pregnancy that may result in adverse health effects. Kangaude et al. posit that adolescent pregnancy and childbearing have adverse health and social effects on adolescent girls [24]. Therefore, Lesotho as a state party to CRC has committed itself to facilitate access to contraception for the adolescents in order to protect and improve their health, although the convention does not precisely refer to gender- and social-inclusion considerations.

2.4 Convention on the rights of persons with disabilities

The Convention on the Rights of Persons with Disabilities (CRPD) enjoins states parties to recognise that persons with disabilities (PWDs) have the right to the enjoyment of the highest attainable standard of health without discrimination on the basis of disability. Thus, article 25 provides that states parties should ensure access to gender-sensitive health services which include sexual and reproductive health services to persons with disabilities. However, the Committee on the Rights of Persons with Disabilities Draft General Comment No. 3 of 2016 notes that women with disabilities are denied access to information related to contraception and family planning because they are assumed to be asexual, yet they have the right to choose the number and spacing of their children like all women. Moreover, children with disabilities lack access of a full range of appropriate and freely chosen contraceptives; as a result, adolescent girls with disabilities experience unwanted pregnancies and sexually transmitted infections [25].

It has been noted that Lesotho has ratified CRPD; therefore, it is obligated to provide adolescents with disabilities with access to gender-sensitive contraception. Thus, the expectation is that this provision of the CRPD is reflected in the health-related legislation, policies, guidelines and practices of the Kingdom of Lesotho. Nevertheless, there are also some gaps identified in the convention: PWDs have been stated as a homogeneous group in the convention. As a result, literacy issues and geographic locations of other people with disabilities have been ignored by the convention.

2.5 Protocol to the African charter on human and peoples' rights on the rights of women in Africa

Under the African human rights system, Lesotho has ratified the African Charter on Human and Peoples' Rights (Banjul Charter) and African Charter on Human and Peoples' Rights and Protocol to the African Charter on Human and Peoples' Rights on the Rights of Women in Africa (Maputo Protocol). The Banjul Charter is silent on contraception or sexual and reproductive health; nevertheless, article 14 of the Maputo Protocol focuses on sexual and reproductive rights of women in Africa. Article 14 binds states parties to ensure that the right to sexual and reproductive health of women is respected and promoted, including the right to choose any method of contraception, control fertility, have family planning education and decide whether to have children, the number of children and the spacing of children. Accordingly, Maziwisa argues that article 14 of the Maputo Protocol protects the rights of adolescent girls to family planning education, controlling their fertility by deciding whether to have children, the number and spacing of children and choosing any method of contraception [see 18]. Maziwisa further states that Maputo Protocol obligates states to ensure that they protect adolescent girls against sexually transmitted infections such as HIV and AIDS and stay informed about their own or partners' health status, especially if they are infected with sexually transmitted infections.

In addition, Maziwisa asserts that article 14(2) enjoins states to take appropriate measures geared towards providing enough, affordable and accessible sexual and reproductive health and rights education in rural areas. The cost of contraception services and methods may be too costly for adolescents, thereby prohibiting them from accessing contraceptives [26]. Therefore, Lesotho has committed itself to provide adolescent girls with affordable and accessible sexual and reproductive health and rights and education in the rural areas. On the other hand, Maputo Protocol does not have provisions for adolescent boys and specific provisions for adolescents with disabilities. Thus, the protocol does not entail contraception issues for adolescents through the gender- and social-inclusion lens, thereby leaving gaps for binding Lesotho to ensure equitable access to contraception for adolescent girls and boys, even though it could be argued that the protocol is gender-specific – it is focusing on women only in Africa.

3. Domestic laws for adolescents' access to contraception in Lesotho

This section entails constitutional provisions and other statutory provisions that link access to contraception for adolescents, and they shall be linked in conformity with international norms.

3.1 Constitution of Lesotho

Sexual and reproductive health rights of adolescents, including a right to contraception, are enshrined in the Constitution of 1993, which provides that every citizen has fundamental human rights and freedoms. Section 27(1)(a) provides that Lesotho shall adopt policies aimed at ensuring the highest attainable standard of physical and mental health for its citizens, including policies designed to reduce stillbirth rate and infant mortality rate and improve health development of the child. Thus, adolescents are citizens of Lesotho, and they have a right to health, including contraception. However, the right to health is non-justiciable because it is a socio-economic right in the Constitution of Lesotho. The right to health is closely related to and dependent on the realisation of the right to life [27]. 'Therefore, violation of the right to health is concurrently a violation of the right to inherent life' [28]. Moreover, the case of *International Pen and others (On behalf of Ken Saro-Wiwa) v Nigeria* links the right to health to the right to life [29]. The right to life is provided in Section 5 of the Constitution. Shah and Ahman assert that unwanted pregnancy is a serious risk to the life, survival and development of adolescents in Africa [30], thereby necessitating protection of life by ensuring that children avoid unwanted pregnancy and have access to contraception (see [24]).

Section 18 of the Constitution prohibits discrimination, and Section 18(2) provides that no person shall be treated in a discriminatory manner by any person acting by virtue of any written law or in the performance of the functions of any public office or any public authority. Kangaude et al. assert that non-discrimination means that health-care providers should not discriminate against minor girls in terms of access to contraceptives; moreover, states should be aware of intersectional discrimination in terms of age, gender and disability (see [24]). It seems that the Constitution does not discriminate between adolescents against access to contraception from the gender- and social-inclusion perspective, though it is not explicitly stated.

Furthermore, Section 14(1) provides for the freedom of expression for every person, including freedom to receive ideas and information without interference. According to UN Committee on the Rights of the Child (CRC) General comment No. 15 (2013) on the right of the child to the enjoyment of the highest attainable standard of health (art. 24), 17 April 2013, CRC/C/GC/15, children should express their views on accessing and using contraception, as well as their experience of the quality of care [31]. Therefore, health-care providers should provide appropriate information to adolescents in a manner that respects their level of maturity and engage the adolescents in decision-making according to their evolving capacities [32]. Section 14(1) of the Constitution of Lesotho protects different groups of adolescents against violation of the freedom to receive information about contraception and express their opinions about contraceptive services they receive. Therefore, the Constitution implicates access to contraception for adolescents using the gender- and social-inclusion lens because it makes a provision for freedom to receive information for every Mosotho.

3.2 Children's protection and welfare act 2011

Section 6 of the Children's Protection and Welfare Act of 2011 (CPWA) makes a provision of protecting adolescents against any form of discrimination on the basis of sex, disability or socio-economic status. Therefore, CPWA provides for equal access to contraception for adolescents where such services are available. In addition, Section 11(1) and (6) of the act upholds children's rights to access to sexual and reproductive health information appropriate to their age. Thus, the act provides for access to contraception information for adolescents. On the other hand, the enforcement of this law is a challenge [33]. Nevertheless, the act does not have provisions in terms of gender equality and social inclusion so as to ensure equal access to contraception information. As a result, disadvantaged and marginalised adolescents are excluded from being protected by the aforementioned section of the CPWA. It has also been noted that the act is silent on access to contraception.

4. Administrative measures for providing contraception

This section provides details about administrative measures taken by the state to ensure that there is access to contraception. The measures will be analysed by looking into adolescents' access to contraception from gender- and social-inclusion perspective.

4.1 Lesotho health policy 2011

The objective of the Lesotho Health Policy of 2011 is to make pregnancy and childbirth safe for mothers and newborns and reproductive health services acceptable to individuals, families and communities. The policy measures include:

- Ensuring access to safe, effective, affordable and acceptable reproductive health services including family-planning services to youth, women and men.

- Promoting and enhancing adolescent sexual and reproductive health, including prevention of transmission of HIV and other STIs.

This policy facilitates adolescents' access to contraception where it makes reference to ensuring access to family-planning services to youth and promoting and enhancing adolescent sexual and reproductive health. However, the policy is gender-blind because it does not clarify gender considerations linked to adolescents in terms of access to contraception. Furthermore, social-inclusion issues such as considering access to contraception in the rural areas and for adolescents with disabilities have not been part of the policy.

4.2 Village health Programme policy 2020

The Village Health Programme Policy's mission is to have equitable access to quality health services. Assumably, quality health services include sexual and reproductive health services that include equitable access to contraception for adolescents. Furthermore, one of the guiding principles of the policy is gender sensitivity and responsiveness, as well as special consideration of women because of their special reproductive role. The objectives of the policy include to extend health-care coverage to all citizens of Lesotho, including people with disabilities and people living in remote, rural and hard to reach parts of the country.

The policy generalises facilitation of equitable access to health-care services at the community level with a specific objective on inclusive health-care services. However, the policy is silent on adolescents as a group; they are assumed to be part of the society eligible for access to health-care services at the community level. Moreover, the policy is silent on access to sexual and reproductive health services, and therefore, it does not have policy objectives or strategic actions on access to contraception for adolescents. Thus, the Village Health Programme Policy of 2020 is not gender-responsive or socially inclusive for advancing access to contraception for adolescents at the community level.

4.3 National Family Planning Guidelines for health service providers 2017

The guidelines state that it is crucial to ensure that adolescents have access to youth-friendly contraceptive information, services and counselling in Lesotho. Furthermore, the guidelines provide that all individuals have a right to access to sexual and reproductive services, regardless of their gender or sexual orientation, marital status, age, religious or political beliefs, ethnicity or disability or any other characteristics which could make individuals prone to discrimination. In addition, one of the general guiding principles of these guidelines is that 'family planning services should be made available to all who need them, including adolescents, men and people with disabilities and special needs'. Lastly, there is a specific section about adolescents, including adolescents with disabilities, in the National Family Planning Guidelines for Health Service Providers.

The National Family Planning Guidelines for Health Service Providers guide health-care service providers to provide equitable and inclusive contraceptive services to adolescents, using a gender- and social-inclusion lens because the guidelines do not regard adolescents as a homogenous group. Therefore, these guidelines are responsive to the needs of adolescents in terms of access to contraception in Lesotho.

4.4 National Strategic Development Plan II

One of the strategic objectives of the National Strategic Development Plan II (NSDP II) 2018–2023 is to increase access, coverage and effectiveness of quality health-care service delivery for all by providing universal access to sexual and reproductive health-care services to all people, with a focus on adolescents, youth and other vulnerable groups. Thus, NSDP II plans to promote equitable and inclusive access to contraception to adolescents because it singles out adolescents and other vulnerable groups.

4.5 Lesotho gender and development policy 2018: 2023

The objective of this policy is to ensure access to health services to different groups of people of all ages and encourage male involvement in sexual and reproductive health issues. Furthermore, its strategic actions are to promote quality health for all regardless of gender or sexual orientation and provide a wide range of family planning methods and contraceptive options. The Lesotho Gender and Development Policy is not adolescent-responsive because it does not address adolescents' sexual and reproductive health issues from the gender perspective – it is silent about adolescents as a group. Apart from that, the policy is also silent about access to contraception for adolescents.

4.6 National Adolescent Health Policy 2006

The National Adolescent Health Policy of 2006 points out that male adolescents who herd animals are more likely to have their rights violated than other adolescents. Moreover, through this policy, the Government of Lesotho commits itself to ensure that quality sexual and reproductive health services are available to all adolescents, and objective 4 of the policy is to reduce the levels of unwanted pregnancies among adolescents by raising the contraceptive use in sexually active adolescents by 20%.

The policy identifies male adolescents having barriers to access to sexual and reproductive services, thereby not having access to contraception. Therefore, this part is gender-sensitive. On the other hand, the target of 20% is not sex-disaggregated or disaggregated by social groups.

4.7 Empirical findings

Lesotho Demographic and Health Survey of 2014 shows that 79.9% of sexually active females aged 15–19 years were not using any contraception. It also shows pregnancy and pregnancy-related deaths that cause mortality for married and unmarried girls between the ages of 15 and 19 in Lesotho. According to 2016 Population and Housing Census Report of Lesotho, teenage pregnancy is as follows in Lesotho (**Table 1**).

In addition to the findings of the Population and Housing Census Report, the Lesotho Multiple Indicator Cluster Survey 2018 shows that adolescent birth rate[1] is 59 in the urban areas and 114 in the rural areas; in ecological zones, it is 77 in the lowlands, 163 in the foothills, 114 in the mountains and 91 in the Senqu River Valley. Furthermore, the survey shows that the percentage of male adolescents aged 15–19 years who have fathered a live birth is 0.4% for both urban and rural areas.

The three reports show that there is high teenage pregnancy in Lesotho, and this implies that adolescents are still debarred from having access to contraception. Moreover, there are some identified gender gaps and social-exclusion issues in terms of access to contraception for adolescents. The surveys did not capture information on adolescents and contraception using a gender lens or focus on social inclusion issues. This shows that administrative measures to facilitate access to contraception for adolescents are not gender-responsive and integrating social inclusivity. Accordingly, the CEDAW Committee recommended Lesotho to target adolescent girls and boys with special attention to early pregnancy and the control of STIs by providing them with sexual and reproductive health education.

Age	Percentage (%)
13	0.1
14	0.5
15	1.6
16	6.3
17	15.3
18	29.4
19	46.9

Source: 2016 Population and Hosing Census Report of Lesotho.

Table 1.
Teenage pregnancy in Lesotho.

[1] Adolescent birth rate is the number of births to women aged 15–19 years

5. Conclusion

It has been found that Lesotho is a state party to different treaties which bind it to promote access to contraception for adolescents from the gender- and social-inclusion perspective, though some treaties are not gender-specific. Thus, Lesotho facilitates access to contraception for adolescents from the gender- and social-inclusion perspective in respect of international law, and this has barriers to implementation because provisions of treaties are only justiciable in Lesotho if they have been domesticated.

The Constitution of Lesotho implicates equitable access to contraception for adolescents from the gender- and social-inclusion perspective because the Constitution provides for gender sensitive and inclusive access to information on sexual and reproductive health. Nevertheless, the Children's Protection and Welfare Act does not have provisions on gender equality and social inclusion so as to ensure equal access to contraception information for adolescents. As a result, disadvantaged and marginalised adolescents are excluded from being protected by the law with respect to right to access to contraception. The act is also silent on access to contraception.

Administratively, National Family Planning Guidelines for Health Service Providers of 2017 and National Strategic Development Plan II are the only strategies which are gender-responsive and use social-inclusion lens to facilitate access to contraception for adolescents. Other policies are gender-blind and silent on adolescents and access to contraception. Lastly, empirical findings show that many adolescents do not have access to contraception, and gender- and social-inclusion issues are not taken into consideration where adolescents may have access to contraception. Therefore, concerted efforts of different stakeholders are required for advancing adolescents' access to contraception from a gender- and social-inclusion perspective in order to enhance universal access to contraception by adolescents in Lesotho.

Author details

Mathoka Khaile[1,2]

1 University of Pretoria, South Africa

2 Lesotho Nutrition and Health System Strengthening Project, Ministry of Health, Lesotho, South Africa

*Address all correspondence to: mkhaile2014@gmail.com

References

[1] Tuoane M, Diamond I, Madise N. Use of family planning in Lesotho: The importance of quality of care and access. African Population Studies. 2015;**18**(2):107

[2] World Health Organisation. Medical Eligibility Criteria for Contraceptive Use. 5th ed. World Health Organisation; 2015. Available from: https://www.who.int

[3] Todd NJ, Black AY. Contraception for adolescents. Journal of Clinical Research in Pediatric Endocrinology. 2020;**12910**:28-40

[4] Lelisa N. Access to Emergency Contraception among Adolescent Girls in Lesotho [Thesis]. Pretoria: University of Pretoria; 2016

[5] Cook R, Dickens BM. Recognising adolescents evolving capacities to exercise choice in reproductive healthcare. International Journal of Gynaecology and Obstetrics. 2000;**70**:13

[6] Mabele M. Determinants of Contraceptive Use among Young Women in Lesotho [Thesis]. Durban: University of Kwazulu-Natal; 2010

[7] Nwankwo BO, Nwoke EA. Risky sexual behaviours among adolescents in Owerri municipal: Predictors of unmet family health needs. African Journal of Reproductive Health. 2009;**13**:234

[8] UNESCO. Young People Today, Time to Act Now: Why Adolescents and Young People Need Comprehensive Sexuality Education and Sexual and Reproductive Health Services in Eastern and Southern Africa. UNESCO, Report; 2013. p. 8. Available from: https://healtheducationalresources.unesco.org

[9] Babatunde OA et al. Contraception among students of public secondary schools in Ilorin, Nigeria. Pan African Medical Journal. 2016;**23**:74. DOI: 10.11604/pamj.2016.23.74.8688

[10] Madkour AS et al. Early adolescent sexual initiation as a problem behaviour: A comparative study of five nations. Journal of Adolescents Health. 2010;**47**(4):389-398

[11] Matope FB. An Assessment of Factors That Determine Usage of Contraceptive Services among Adolescent Women in Lesotho: An Analytical Cross-Sectional Study of Maseru City Secondary School Students [Thesis]. Cape Town: University of Western Cape; 2022

[12] Savage- Oyekunle OA. Adolescents' access to emergency contraception in Africa: An empty promise? African Human Rights Law Journal. 2018;**17**:470

[13] Gurung R et al. The burden of adolescent motherhood and health consequences in Nepal. Pregnancy and Childbirth. 2020;**20**:2

[14] WHO. Adolescent Sexual and Reproductive Health and Rights. Barometer. Vol. 5. WHO; 2020. Available from: https://www.who.int

[15] Centre for Reproductive Rights. The Right to Contraceptive Information and Services for Women and Adolescents. Centre for Reproductive Rights, Briefing Paper.; 2010. pp. 6-7. Available from: https://reproductiverights.org

[16] Cislaghi B, Shakya H. Social norms and adolescents' sexual health: An introduction for practitioners working in low and mid-income African countries. African Journal Reproductive Health. 2018;**22**:38

[17] Cislaghi B, Heise L. Gender norms and social norms: Differences,

similarities and why they matter in prevention science. Sociology of Health & Illness. 2020;**42**:407

[18] Maziwisa MR. Barriers to access to contraceptives for adolescent girls in Zimbabwe as a human rights challenge. In: Durojaye E, Mirugi-Mukundi G, Ngwena C, editors. Advancing Sexual and Reproductive Health and Rights in Africa: Constraints and Opportunities. London: Routledge; 2021. pp. 67-70

[19] Cook R. International human rights and women's reproductive health. Studies in Family Planning. 1993;**24**(2):73-79

[20] CEDAW/C/LSO/CO. Committee on the Elimination of Discrimination against Women Concluding Observations of the Committee on the Elimination of Discrimination against Women Lesotho. CEDAW/C/LSO/CO; 2011. Available from: https://www2.ohchr.org/bodies/cedaw/docs

[21] Culwell KR, Vekemans M, de Silva U, Hurwitz M. Critical gaps in universal access to reproductive health: Contraception and prevention of unsafe abortion. International Journal of Gynaecology and Obstetrics. 2010;**110**:13

[22] Durojaye E. Access to contraception for adolescents in Africa: A human rights challenge. Comparative International Law Journal of Southern Africa. 2011;**44**(1):1

[23] Bearinger LH, Sieving RE, Ferguson J, Sharma V. Global perspectives on the sexual and reproductive health of adolescents: Patterns, prevention and potential. The Lancet. 2007;**369**:1220-1231

[24] Kangaude GD, Macleod C, Coast E, Fetters T. Integrating child rights standards in contraceptive and abortion care for minors in Africa. International Journal of Gynaecology and Obstetrics. 2022;**158**(3):998-1004

[25] Assefa N et al. Reported barriers to healthcare access and service disruptions caused by COVID-19 in Burkina Faso, Ethiopia and Nigeria: A telephone survey. The American Journal of Tropical Medicine and Hygiene. 2021;**105**(2):323-330

[26] Todd N, Black A. Contraception for adolescents. Journal of Clinical Research in Paediatrics. 2020;**12**:28-29

[27] CESCR General Comment 14 UN Doc E/C.12/2000/4 para 21

[28] Khaile M. Access to Emergency Contraception for Rape Survivors in Lesotho [Thesis]. Pretoria: University of Pretoria; 2019

[29] International Pen and others (On behalf of Ken Saro-Wiwa) v Nigeria

[30] Shah IH, Ahman E. Unsafe abortion differentials in 2008 by age and developing country region: High burden among young women. Reproductive Health Matters. 2012;**20**:170

[31] UN Committee on the Rights of the Child (CRC) General comment No. 15 on the right of the child to the enjoyment of the highest attainable standard of health (art. 24). 2013. CRC/C/GC/15

[32] Coughlin KW. Medical decision-making in paediatrics: Infancy to adolescence. Paediatrics & Child Health. 2018;**23**(2):138

[33] Shale I. Sexual and reproductive rights of women with disabilities: Implementing international human rights standards in Lesotho. In: African Disability Rights Book. Vol. 3. Pretoria, South Africa: University of Pretoria; 2015. p. 45

Chapter 2

Adolescents, Social Media and Access to Reproductive Health Information and Services in Ghana: Prospects and Challenges

Rahma Salifu and Abdulai Abubakari

Abstract

Social media is one of the variables affecting sexual behavior among teenagers in today's society. This study was conducted in Tamale, Ghana, to examine adolescents' application of social media to access and use reproductive health services. The study involved 342 adolescents randomly selected from multicultural and diverse backgrounds of students drawn from four Senior High Schools in the Tamale metropolis of the Northern Region. Data was collected using semi-structured questionnaires and interview guides. The quantitative data were analyzed using STATA 16.0, chi-square test of association, and binary logistic regression at a 5% significance level. The study found that 45.4% of adolescents accessed reproductive health (RH) information through social media. The study showed that there was a significant association between using a mobile phone to access RH information and romantic relationship ($p < 0.001$), awareness of reproductive health ($p < 0.040$), respondents' place of residence ($p < 0.040$) and occupation of guardian ($p < 0.040$), mobile phone ownership ($p < 0.004$), social media use ($p < 0.001$), means of accessing RH using a mobile phone ($p < 0.02$) and whether their problem was solved ($p < 0.001$). The study concludes that, despite the high utilization of social media and awareness of reproductive health services, less than half (45.4%) of the adolescents use social media by adolescents to access adolescent reproductive health services in the Tamale metropolis.

Keywords: adolescents, social media, reproductive health service, knowledge, sexually transmitted infections

1. Introduction

The new digital media field has changed how young people obtain information and interact with one another [1]. Computer-mediated systems which allow individuals and communities to connect, interact, link and share content are known as "social media" Field [2]. Social media initiatives can instantly reach bigger followers via recognizable venues, using social networks' credibility and impact [3]. Social media platforms are constantly changing [4], as a result, young people are increasingly communicating online instead of in person, and smartphones can obstruct face-to-face conversations adolescent females are avid users of social media as compared to boys, are more vulnerable to cyberbullying, and are more likely to suffer from mental health issues [5].

Approximately half the global population possesses a mobile phone, and 42% access the Internet Okeleke [6]. Peer pressure and unpleasant behaviors, such as cyberbullying, internet fraud, pornography, computer or cell phone gaming, video gaming are some of the few examples that social media can have adverse effects on adolescents' self-perception as well as interpersonal connections [5]. In the United States in 2014, 81% of 12–17 years used social media. Internet connectivity and social media use by young people in low- and middle-income nations are growing, although not to the exact extent as in high-income one's [3].

Social media platform is one of the variables affecting sexual behavior among teenagers in today's society. Using these platforms has positive and harmful effects on adolescents, particularly regarding sexual content. They learn through watching individual interactions displayed on these platforms and then assimilating them, notably when their personalities are recognized or seem spared from the consequences of their actions [7].

According to Jumia's Annual Mobile Report 2018, Ghana is one of the top mobile markets in Africa, with 34.57 million users and a subscriber base of 119%. (www.ghanaweb.com). According to a study by international digital organizations. We Are Social, and Hootsuite, Ghana has 5.6 million active social media users, 19.53 million phone users, and 9.28 million active wireless internet clients, making up 32% of the country's population. (www.businessworldghana.com).

Most teenagers prefer to be alone at this age rather than share time with their parents and family. Due to this, most parents find it challenging to hold conversations with their children. As a result, they get much of their sexual information from colleagues, friends, and social media. Adolescent interaction is most productive when it occurs within a client-therapist relationship that is transparent and nonjudgmental, fosters trust and mental comfort, and provides a sense of involvement and liberty [8].

Adolescents even have social media mentors as artists, actors, broadcasters, and entertainers. Those influencers frequently share details about their private lives, fashion choices, and views on sexual topics on social networks. Adolescents can be greatly affected by culture and the surrounding environment. As a result, adolescents pick up information from their surroundings. Their sexual behaviors are influenced by their mimicking or emulating sexual actions on social media. Adolescents acquire sexual practices including the frequency of sex depicted as appropriate on social media, several sex partners, casual sex partners, and contraception.

Social media users may be susceptible to concerns such as inaccurate self-diagnosis, decreased personal interaction, dependency, probable privacy violations, insecurities, and anxiety [9, 10]. Despite these obstacles, numerous studies have shown positive impacts linked with social media utilization, such as availability of information, support availability through online support groups, drive, and personal worth [11, 12].

Several studies have been conducted in Ghana on adolescent reproductive health information, service, and associated factors. An investigation was undertaken to evaluate the perception level and point out the main factors of measuring the standard of care [13]. A study on adolescent reproductive health to assess the influencing factors, education and the usage of reproductive health facilities indicates that 85% had the knowledge sexually transmitted infections as the prevailing issue, with 78% and 50% of adolescents had gone through reproductive health education [14].

DOI: http://dx.doi.org/10.5772/intechopen.111768

Adolescents experience mental, physical, physiological and mental challenges that affect their developmental and productive potential. Girls forced into undesirable relationships or marriages become victims of unsafe abortions, unintended pregnancies, high-risk childbirth, STDs, and even HIV. A study conducted in Yong Dakpemyili shows that 37% of pregnant adolescents have abortions, 11% go through cesarean section during delivery, 8.9% are stillborn and 7% have early neonatal mortality Field [15]. Adolescents frequently lack knowledge about sexually transmitted infections (STIs), pregnancy, HIV/AIDS screening and treatment, and other reproductive health issues, all serious health concerns in Ghana. As a result, the country's progress toward achieving Sustainable Development Goal 3 is hampered.

By the District Health Information Management System of Ghana Health Service, from 2016 to 2020, there are 555,575 adolescent pregnancies in Ghana; 13 teenage pregnancies were recorded each hour, and 110,000 were recorded in 2020. Despite the prospect of social media in disseminating juvenile sexual and reproductive information, this has not been explored in Ghana. For instance, there needs to be more research on how adolescents utilize social media to seek resources for reproductive health. In the Tamale metropolis, more study is required on this subject. Against this backdrop, this study aims to assess the contribution of social media usage in adolescent reproductive health services and information in the Tamale metropolis.

2. Theoretical framework

The Unified Theory of Acceptance and Use of Technology (UTAUT) serves as the theoretical foundation for this study. The need to employ technological innovation is influenced by performance expectations, effort expectations, and social influence [16]. The theory is renowned for examining the moderating impact of user demographics on the link between social media variables and user behavioral intention. This theory is an integration of eight other crucial theories, such as the Technology Acceptance Model (TAM) by [17], the Model of Personal Computer Utilization (MPCU) by Varela et al. [18], the Innovation Diffusion Theory (IDT) by Rogers [19], the Theory of Reasoned Action (TRA) by Fishbein and Ajzen [20], the Motivational Model (MM) by Davis et al. [21], the Theory of Planned Behavior (TPB) by Ajzen [22], Social Cognitive Theory (SCT) by Compeau and Higgins [23], and finally a Combined TAM-TPB (C-TAM-TPB) by Taylor and Todd [24]. It is crucial to note that UTAUT is shown to be a better acceptable predictor of the chance of technology innovation success after a thorough analysis of other reliable models [25]. UTAUT aids in a better understanding of the factors that influence adolescents' adoption of technology, who are notoriously aggressive and engaged in pursuing sexual and reproductive options. UTAUT is the preferred theoretical framework for this study because it has four aims. The Unified Theory of Acceptance and Use of Technology (UTAUT) is formulated after empirically examining the existing users' acceptance models and confronting the eight models described above. It is then validated. It is crucial to remember that sociocultural influences play a role in the social media usage of adolescents in Ghana. According to the theory, individual intentions to employ technological innovation are influenced by social influence, effort, expectations, and performance. Social media offer adolescents the space mentioned above. Peer influence, coupled with their youthful exuberance and desire to try new things, found expression in social media, which meets their expectations. The theory is well recognized for examining the moderating effect of user demographics on the association between social media factors and user behavioral intention. UTAUT was chosen for this study because it is a more accurate predictor of the likelihood that technological advances will succeed [25]. UTAUT provides the required philosophical underpinning to understand the factors that influence technology acceptance and adolescents' use of social media to access sexual reproductive information so that the necessary policies can be developed.

3. Methods

3.1 Study setting

Tamale is the official capital town of the Northern Region. It also unofficially doubles as the capital of northern Ghana because it hosts all manner of people across the north and south of Ghana. It is a cosmopolitan settlement and the third-largest city in Ghana. In the past three decades, sporadic and spasmodic eruptions of ethnic, religious, chieftaincy and land conflicts, forced hundreds of people from the hinterlands to migrate to Tamale. The metropolis also has some of the best educational institutions in Ghana; three universities, two colleges of education, two nursing training colleges, about 20 Senior high Schools and more than 200 basic schools. Tamale also has some of the best health facilities, including the Tamale Teaching Hospital, Tamale West Hospital, Central Hospital, SDA Hospital, and many other private hospitals.

Tamale was chosen for the study because it has some of the best socio-economic infrastructure and offers opportunities to many people across the globe. Due to its cosmopolitan nature, it also has cultural diversity and offers a resemblance of miniature Ghanian and global cultures. More importantly, the study dwelled on Senior High Schools (SHS) because most of the adolescents using the social media are concentrated in these schools. Secondly, due to the computerized SHS placement system adopted in Ghana over a decade ago, the SSS comprises students from all over Ghana and from different geographical, religious, cultural and ethnic backgrounds.

3.2 Study population and sampling

Teenagers (10–19) enrolled in senior high schools in Tamale Metropolis were the target population. The formula for a point estimate sample developed by Snedecor and Cochran [26] was used to determine the sample size. In a survey by Marie et al. in 2020, they indicated that about 66.7% of teenagers used social media to look up health-related information. This study also adopted 66.7% proportion of social media usage as the basis.

$$N = Z2\{P\}\{1 - P\} / m^2$$

$$Z(\text{Standard value for } 95\%\text{confidence level}) = 1.96$$

$$P(\text{Proportion of social media usage for ASRHS}) = 66.7\%(0.667)$$

$$m(\text{margin of error}) = 5\%(0.05)$$

$$N = 1.962\{0.667\}\{1 - 0.667\} / 0.052$$

$$N = 3.8416\{0.667\}\{0.333\}/0.0025$$

$$N = 341.3$$

In all, the total sample size was 342 adolescents.

3.3 Sampling technique and procedure

The Tamale Metropolis has eight public senior high schools, including vocational ones. Using a multistage selection strategy, the adolescents for this study were selected for the sample. The first stage involved the simple random selection ('the lotto technique') of the Senior High Schools in the Tamale metropolis. This was to ensure that all the SHS have equal chances of being selected. Thus, four SHS were selected; Ghana Senior High School, St. Charles Seminary, Vitting Senior High and Tamale Girls' Senior High School. The second stage involved sampling adolescents from these schools. A proportionate-to-size sampling approach was used to determine the number of adolescents to be selected from each school. A simple random sampling approach was then used to select students eligible to participate in the study. The eligibility criteria were being an adolescent and having access to a computer or cell phone. Thus, 342 adolescents were selected. In addition, six focus group discussions (FGD) were held in various parts of Tamale; Bamvum, Changli, Zogbeli, Gumani, Dungu and Kpalsi. Two groups were a mixture of boys and girls, another two groups were only boys, and the last two were only girls. The mixed focus groups comprised of eight adolescents, four girls and four boys. The purpose of the FGDs was to get detailed information from the adolescents to complement the survey data (**Table 1**).

3.4 Data collection tools and procedures

Self-administered questionnaires were used for data collection in this study. The questionnaire was the leading tool to gather the data, and it was made of three sections, including sociodemographic characteristics of respondents, knowledge and utilization and the factors influencing adolescent sexual and reproductive health services.

3.5 Data management and statistical analysis

Data collected were entered into Microsoft Excel 2017, cleaned and imported into STATA version 16.0 for analysis. The researchers ensured that participants were

Name of school	Student population	Boys	Girls	Number selected
Ghana Senior High School	1885	976	909	140
St. Charles Seminary	309	309	0	23
Vitting Senior High	1118	792	326	83
Tamale Girls' Senior High School	1300	0	1300	96
Total	4612	2077	2535	342

Table 1.
Proportion of students sampled from selected senior high schools.

taken through the questionnaire to understand each question well. Respondents were also given 2 weeks to return the completed forms. This provided them ample time to respond to all the questions. Categorical variables such as sex, marital status, religion, utilization of services, type of media and the platform used were analyzed and summarized using frequencies and proportions at a 95% Confidence Interval (CI). Quantitative continuous variables such as age were summarized into mean and standard deviation. A chi-square test of association was employed to evaluate the relationship between the result variable and the different variables. The chi-square analysis's level of significance was set at 5%. At a significance threshold of 5%, a crude and adjusted binary logistic regression was employed to assess the strength of the correlation between the outcome variable and the numerous variables.

4. Results

4.1 Sociodemographic characteristics of the study participants

Of the 342 students studied, 98.3% were between 15 and 19. About two-thirds of the students were females. More than half (57.0%) reside in urban areas. The majority, 95.3%, were single in terms of marital status. The occupation of their parents or guardians, most of them were traders. Most of the students were from the second year (**Table 2**).

4.2 Study participants reproductive health characteristics

More than one-third of the respondents (40.6%) were in a romantic relationship, and 86.8% mentioned they were not sexually active at the time of the study. Their awareness of reproductive health services, almost all (93.9%) were aware of the services, with the majority of the respondents (85.7%) getting their source from schools (**Table 3**).

4.3 Social media utilization among study participants

On their access to social media, when asked about the ownership of mobile phones, more than two-thirds (76.9%) answered affirmatively, 51.5% accessed social media, and 71.2% mentioned Facebook as the most frequently used social media. On how often they visited social media, the majority 74.3% said sometimes. The majority of the respondents (69.6%) preferred accessing reproductive health services via social media, and most of them stated that the problem for which they accessed social media reproductive services was solved after accessing it (**Table 4**).

4.4 Accessing reproductive health information through social media

Out of the 342 students studied, 45.4% 95%CI (40.0–51.0) indicated they have ever accessed reproductive health information through social media (**Figure 1**).

4.5 Sociodemographic characteristics of the participants, Tamale Metropolis, 2022

The Chi-square analysis showed that respondents' place of residence ($p < 0.040$) and occupation of guardian ($p < 0.040$) were significantly associated with accessing reproductive health information via social media (**Table 5**).

Characteristics	Frequency (N)	Percentage (%)
Age group (years)		
10–14	6	1.75
15–19	336	98.25
Sex		
Female	235	68.71
Male	107	31.29
Religion		
Christianity	95	27.78
Islam	247	72.22
Marital status		
Single	322	95.27
Married	5	1.48
Cohabiting	11	3.25
Residence		
Rural	147	42.98
Urban	195	57.02
Education		
SHS Form 1	1	0.29
SHS Form 2	293	85.67
SHS Form 3	48	14.04
Occupation of guardian		
Farmer	108	32.34
Government employee	74	22.16
Trader	140	41.92
Others	12	3.59

Table 2.
Sociodemographic characteristics of the study participants.

Characteristics	Frequency (N)	Percentage (%)
Romantic relationship		
No	203	59.36
Yes	139	40.64
Sexually active		
No	296	86.80
Yes	45	13.20
Awareness of RH		
No	21	6.14
Yes	321	93.86

Characteristics	Frequency (N)	Percentage (%)
Information source		
Family members	13	4.05
School	275	85.67
Friends	6	1.87
Media	9	2.80
Religious gathering	5	1.56
Health provider	13	4.05

Table 3.
Study participants reproductive health characteristics.

Characteristics	Frequency (N)	Percentage (%)
Phone ownership		
No	79	23.10
Yes	263	76.90
Social media use		
No	166	48.54
Yes	176	51.46
Media frequently used		
Facebook	111	71.15
Instagram	12	7.69
Twitter	4	2.56
YouTube	29	18.59
Frequency of use		
Always	23	15.13
Rarely	16	10.53
sometimes	113	74.34
Preference for accessing RH		
Physical	92	30.36
Social media	211	69.64
Means of access		
Communication App	39	14.89
Text (SMS)	86	32.82
Video call	12	4.58
Voice call	18	6.87
Websites	107	40.84
Problem solved		
No	53	21.54
Yes	193	78.46

Table 4.
Social media utilization among study participants, tamale metropolis.

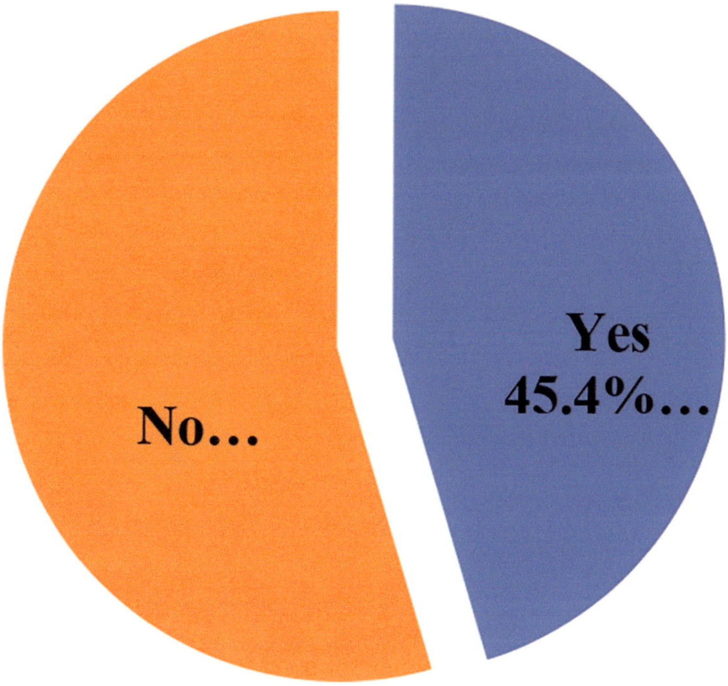

Figure 1.
Accessing reproductive health information through social media, Tamale Metropolis. Chi-square test of Association between accessing RH using social media and.

Characteristics	Social media to access RH			
	No	Yes	÷2	P-value
Age group (years)			1.321	0.250
10–14	4 (80.0%)	1 (20.0%)		
15–19	180 (54.22%)	152 (45.78%)		
Sex			3.444	0.063
Female	134 (58.01%)	97 (41.99%)		
Male	50 (47.17%)	56 (52.83%)		
Religion			1.557	0.212
Christianity	57 (60.00%)	38 (40.00%)		
Islam	127 (52.48%)	115 (47.52)		
Marital status			2.211	0.331
Cohabiting	7 (70.00%)	3 (30.00%)		
Married	4 (80.00%)	1 (20.00%)		
Single	184 (55.26%)	149 (44.74%)		
Residence			4.203	0.040**
Rural	89 (60.96%)	57 (39.04%)		
Urban	95 (49.74%)	96 (50.26%)		

Characteristics	Social media to access RH			
	No	Yes	÷2	P-value
Education			1.256	0.534
SHS Form 1	0	1 (100.00%)		
SHS Form 2	157 (54.51%)	131 (45.49%)		
SHS Form 3	27 (56.25%)	21 (43.75%)		
Occupation of guardian			8.289	0.040**
Farmer	69 (65.09%)	37 (34.91%)		
Government employee	31 (43.66%)	40 (56.34%)		
Trader	75 (53.57%)	65 (46.43%)		
Others	6 (50.00%)	6 (50.00%)		

Chi-square test of Association between accessing RH using social media and sociodemographic characteristics of the participants.

Table 5.
Bivariate analysis of the association between accessing RH using social media and sociodemographic characteristics of the participants.

4.6 Participants reproductive health characteristics, tamale metropolis

The Chi-square analysis showed that being in a romantic relationship ($p < 0.001$), and having an awareness of reproductive health ($p < 0.040$) were significantly associated with accessing reproductive health services via social media (**Table 6**).

4.7 Social media utilization among study participants, tamale metropolis

The Chi-square analysis showed that respondents' mobile phone ownership ($p < 0.004$), social media use ($p < 0.001$), means of accessing RH using a mobile

Characteristics	Social media to access RH			
	No	Yes	÷2	P-value
Romantic relationship			16.664	0.001**
No	127 (63.82%)	72 (36.18%)		
Yes	57 (41.30%)	81 (58.70%)		
Sexually active			3.751	0.053
No	165 (56.51%)	127 (43.49%)		
Yes	18 (40.91%)	26 (59.09%)		
Awareness of RH			4.212	0.040**
No	16 (76.19%)	5 (23.81%)		
Yes	168 (53.16%)	148 (46.84%)		

Chi-square test of Association between accessing RH using Social Media and participants' reproductive health characteristics.

Table 6.
Bivariate analysis of association between accessing RH using social media and participants' reproductive health characteristics.

phone ($p < 0.02$) and whether their problem was solved ($p < 0.001$) were significantly associated with accessing reproductive health services via social media among the study participants (**Table 7**).

4.8 Factors associated with using social media to access reproductive health services

Male students were more likely than female students to use social media to get reproductive health services, with a difference of 62%. (aOR = 1.62, 95% CI 1.01–2.59). Students who resided in urban areas had 55% higher odds of accessing reproductive health services via social media than their rural dwelling colleagues (aOR = 1.55, 95% CI 1.00–2.41). On their relationship status, students who were in a romantic relationship had 2.3 times increased odds of accessing reproductive health services via social media compared to their colleagues who were not in any romantic relationship (aOR = 2.25, 95% CI 1.39–3.64,). Among students who use social media,

Characteristics	Social Media to access RH			
	No	Yes	÷2	P-value
Phone ownership			8.155	0.004**
No	53 (68.83%)	24 (31.17%)		
Yes	131 (50.38%)	129 (49.62%)		
Social media use			53.974	0.001**
No	122 (75.31%)	40 (24.69%)		
Yes	62 (35.43%)	113 (64.57%)		
Media frequently used			2.374	0.498
Facebook	35 (31.82%)	75 (68.18%)		
Instagram	6 (50.00%)	6 (50.00%)		
Twitter	1 (25.00%)	3 (75.00%)		
YouTube	12 (41.38%)	17 (58.62%)		
Preference for accessing RH			2.147	0.143
Physical	50 (56.18%)	39 (43.82%)		
Social media	99 (46.92%)	112 (53.08%)		
Means of access			12.791	0.012**
Communication App	19 (48.72%)	20 (51.28%)		
Text (SMS)	40 (46.51%)	46 (53.49%)		
Video call	7 (58.33%)	5 (41.67%)		
Voice call	11 (64.71%)	6 (35.29%)		
Websites	32 (29.91%)	75 (70.09%)		
Problem solved			14.058	0.001**
No	32 (60.38%)	21 (39.62%)		
Yes	62 (32.12%)	131 (67.88%)		

Table 7.
Association between accessing RH via social media and social media utilization among study participants.

Characteristics	COR 95%CI	P-value	AOR 95%CI	P-value
Age group (years)				
10–14				
15–19	3.38 (0.37–30.54)	0.279	3.36 (0.37–30.87)	0.284
Sex				
Female				
Male	1.55 (0.97–2.46)	0.064	1.62 (1.01 2.59)	0.045**
Religion				
Christianity				
Islam	1.36 (0.84–2.20)	0.213	1.47 (0.90 2.40)	0.126
Marital status				
Married				
Single	2.30 (0.72–7.39)	0.160	2.03 (0.63 6.61)	0.238
Residence				
Rural				
Urban	1.58 (1.02–2.44)	0.041	1.55 (1.00 2.41)	0.054**
Education				
SHS Form 2				
SHS Form 3	0.93 (0.50–1.71)	0.804	0.93 (0.50 1.73)	0.814
Romantic relationship				
No				
Yes	2.51 (1.61–3.91)	0.001	2.25 (1.39 3.64)	0.001**
Sexually active				
No				
Yes	1.88 (0.99–3.57)	0.055	1.20 (0.60 2.42)	0.601
Awareness of RH				
No				
Yes	2.82 (1.01–7.88)	0.048	2.14 (0.75 6.10)	0.153
Phone ownership				
No				
Yes	2.17 (1.27–3.73)	0.005	2.01 (1.17 3.49)	0.013**
Social media use				
No				
Yes	5.56 (3.46–8.92)	0.001	6.37 (3.68 11.05)	0.001**
Media frequently used				
Messaging apps				
YouTube	0.71 (0.31–1.62)	0.414	1.20 (0.32 4.42)	0.787
Problem resolved				
No				
Yes	3.22 (1.72–6.03)	0.001	3.403 (1.63 7.09)	0.001**

Table 8.
Multivariate analysis of factors associated with using social media to access reproductive health services.

there were 6.37 times increased odds of accessing reproductive health services via social media compared to their colleagues who do not use social media (aOR = 6.37, 95% CI 3.68–11.05) (**Table 8**).

4.9 Prospects and challenges

The prospects of using social media to access reproductive health information is grate. The fact more adolescents are using it means it can survive generations. Secondly, there is wider coverage of internet serves in Ghana. The last point is that there is no restrictions to the use of social media in Ghana.

However, the use of social media to access sexual reproductive health information by adolescents comes with some challenges. The study revealed that it has cost implications as it requires smartphones and data for the internet. The study showed that 89% of adolescents considered this twin cost the main obstacle. Smartphones are costly, and only a few adolescents from well-to-do families can afford them. During the FGDs, it came up strongly that most adolescents' desire to own smartphones compels them to engage in thievery. They claimed that most girls who cannot afford them are also involved in prostitution to be able to acquire and maintain them.

Another challenge frequently mentioned by the respondents is the authenticity of the information they obtained through various social media. They get the information mainly from Tiktok, Instagram, Twitter, Whatsapp, Facebook, as well as Google and Yahoo search engines. Sometimes it is difficult to authenticate the veracity of the information they consume. Over three-quarters of the respondents (87%) claimed that some of the information they get from these sources is unreliable and has cost many complications for most adolescents. During the FGDs, respondents cited examples of girls who got pregnant and complicated their situation by relying on social media information to get rid of their pregnancies.

The third major challenge they cited was time consuming, especially by the students. Adolescents spend a lot of time on the social media at the expense of their studies. They claimed that most adolescents spend 2–3 hours per day on their phones. This affects not only their studies, but also their socialization processes. They indicated that most adolescents are engaged in cybercrimes, fraudulent internet deals, games, and pornography.

5. Discussion

The advent of mHealth is due to the development of mobile communication. mHealth services have the chance to make health promotion, protection and prevention interventions easy to access and may also reduce time and distance [27]. With the fast development of mobile communication, there has been a rush in a study into the health advantages of mobile phone use. Experts from various academic fields have been researching popular social media platforms like WhatsApp, Twitter, and Facebook in light of today's culture, including the issues they raise for politics, interpersonal relationships, the general welfare of society, and mental health. With the development of digital and mobile technology, people are now more able than ever to engage in extensive engagement; as a result, a new media era has emerged, having interaction at the core of new media activities.

This study accessed Tamale Metropolis's teenage reproductive health services and information via social media. According to the report, less than half of the teens in the survey had ever used social media to acquire knowledge or services related to reproductive health. This shows that even though teens in the Tamale metropolitan use social media frequently, less than 50% use it to find resources for their reproductive health.

This aligns with research from the Internet and American Life Project at the Pew Research Center, which found that an estimated 30% of youth use social media to learn about health-related topics. This, however, conflicts with the results of a study done in Nigeria with 1800 girls randomly chosen from 18 public senior secondary schools in Lagos State, where social media was the least reliable source of information or services on reproductive health [28]. Additionally, although 94.6% of adolescents use social media, only 3.5% said they used it to look for health-related information, according to a survey by Plaisime et al. [29]. Furthermore, most participants in a cross-sectional study in Nigeria stated that social media was the most often used channel for receiving SRH information and services [30]. Additionally, a study conducted in 2015 by González-Ortega, Vicario-Molina, Martnez, and Orgaz shows that 68.4% of teenagers utilize social media for sexual education.

The use of social media will affect how often teenagers use it to receive services related to adolescent reproductive health. Compared to teenagers who do not use social media, those who do are more likely to discover and use reproductive services. This study found that social media is used by half of the teenagers. Paraphs, because the study was conducted in school, where the school authorities restrict students from using, cell phones, that was why only half of them claimed they used cell phones. A much higher proportion was reported in a study conducted in Philadelphia, USA, where 94.6% of teens said they used social media [29]. The inconsistency in findings could be attributed to the disparity in the settings of the studies.

Regarding social media, they frequently visited, most mentioning Facebook. However, this is inconsistent with a study by Plaisime, which reported Instagram as the social media frequency by study participants [29].

Policymakers and organizations participating in adolescent reproductive health services will make better decisions if they know and comprehend adolescents' choices when deciding how to receive reproductive health information and services. This study found that most teenagers would instead use social media to acquire reproductive health information and services than go to reproductive health facilities. When asked why they would not want to attend a health centre for their reproductive health concerns, students in a focus group discussion cited the attitude of the staff members and how others saw the institution. This conclusion is supported by research by Gray et al. [31], which found that the internet and GPs/family doctors were teenagers' primary sources of knowledge on reproductive health (49.1% and 38.9%, respectively). However, this is inconsistent with the findings of a study conducted by Lim et al. [32], where fewer participants reported being comfortable getting information from social media. The disparity in findings could be attributed to the difference in the characteristics of the study participants. Lim et al., [32] studied young people aged 16–29 years, unlike this study, which interviewed adolescents aged 10–19.

A study by Goodyear et al. [33] stated in general, when looking for healthcare information, young people are turning to new technologies, notably social media. According to their research, social media provides extraordinary and unusual opportunities for the young to be educated and know about health. Additionally, it has a great range of effects on behavioral changes regarding health and lifestyle. Furthermore, persons 18–29 years old were shown to be much more likely to use social media sites to seek remedies for health issues. The survey also discovered that joining health groups on social media is simpler than joining traditional health or fitness groups [33]. Texting on cell phones is more frequent among Ghanaian young aged 18–34 than those aged 35 and beyond [34]. Media has long been recognized as a valuable instrument for enhancing health. The World Health Organization (WHO) proposed transferring health-related information via engaging and audio-visual tools in 1986. Following this, digital technology, also called mobile health (mHealth), has emerged as a means for fostering and attaining health. Using a mobile phone to improve healthy behaviors is known as the mHealth [35].

Consequently, mHealth is viewed as having potential since it addresses the challenges of services being out of reach, if not completely inaccessible, for the most vulnerable people and sexual and reproductive health topics being controversial in most societies [36]. According to recent studies, youth support mobile health programs that can raise general health awareness [36]. mHealth is gathering steam as a critical avenue for connecting young people who face numerous obstacles and difficulties in gaining access to adolescent youth-friendly institutions and has been an effective tool for offering young people information on adolescent reproductive health and services [37]. Health may solve this nomad problem by giving young people ongoing access to knowledge and information. In a research conducted in Ghana in 2015, 31% of participants aged 14–18 and 71% of participants aged 19–25 owned a mobile phone, while 77% of those aged 14–18 and 91% of those aged 19–25 had used a cell phone in the previous 4 weeks [38].

Although the potential for government m-health initiatives to improve healthcare in locations with limited resources has received widespread praise, this opportunity has not yet been fulfilled in the execution of large-scale policy [39]. According to a survey, men are more likely than women to use mobile phones, and young people from higher socioeconomic levels are also more likely to purchase and use mobile phones [40]. According to a study by Rokicki [36], mHealth platforms for teenagers have the potential to engage and increase health awareness among teenage girls from all socioeconomic backgrounds, particularly those who are more likely to experience poor sexual and reproductive health outcomes.

According to the study, a statistically significant link exists between having sex and using teen reproductive health services. Males in this study had higher odds of accessing adolescent reproductive health services via social media than their female counterparts. This may be explained by the fact that guys make up most of the study's social media users. The results of a survey by Marie, which showed a statistically significant sex difference in the frequency of Facebook, Twitter, and Instagram usage for reproductive health information and services, are consistent with these findings [29].

Students' residency during school breaks was another factor that significantly influenced the use of social media to access adolescent reproductive health information and services. Students who resided in urban areas during school breaks were found to have higher odds of accessing health information via social media compared to their counterparts who dwelled in rural regions during school breaks. This could be explained by the availability of electricity and internet connectivity in urban settings compared to rural locations.

Another element that was discovered to be connected to teens using social media to seek information on adolescent reproductive health was their relationship status. Comparatively to those who were not in a romantic relationship, adolescents were more likely to receive information about reproductive health.

The type of reproductive health information and services adolescents are interested in depends significantly on how sexually active they are. Adolescents who engage in sexual activities are more inclined to learn about reproductive health than adolescents who are naïve to sexual activity. More than two-thirds of them were found to be inactive sexually, according to the study. It can be inferred that most teenagers had not engaged in sexual activity. This contrasts with the results of a survey conducted by Asare et al. [41], which indicated that 50.4% of young people were sexually active and that 77.3% of them initiated sex after the age of 15.

Individuals' awareness and knowledge about a service influences their engagement or utilization. Adolescents will only use social media to access reproductive health information and services if they are aware of these services and which social media to visit for this information. This study revealed that over 90% of participants were mindful of adolescent reproductive health services. This suggests that most adolescents in the survey know the benefits of adolescent reproductive health. This aligns with the findings of cross-sectional research on reproductive health knowledge and practices among female adolescents in a Mumbai urban slum, where 212 (88%) women were aware that ARHS services were offered [42]. The consistency in findings can be attributed to the urban nature of the settings of these studies. The results of a survey conducted in Oyo state, Nigeria, where just 13.1% of participants were aware of the adolescent reproductive health services; however, contradict this finding [43].

Adolescents' awareness and use of these services will be influenced by the sources of information and services available to them on adolescent reproductive health. Regarding their source of information, the study revealed that the majority cited school as their source of reproductive health information. This could be explained by the fact that all the adolescents studied were second and third-year students who received lectures on adolescent reproductive health in social studies. Knowing that most adolescents obtain information on their reproductive health from schools, it will be essential to introduce courses that teach students the correct information without shying them away. In a similar study, the majority of the respondents, 72.4 per cent, learned about adolescent reproductive health services school staff. Also, most believed that adolescent sexual and reproductive services and information were critical for young people [44]. This consistency in findings could be attributed to the fact that both studies were conducted among adolescents in secondary schools.

The judgmental nature of health care providers at our health facilities is a critical factor that shies adolescents from accessing reproductive health services. Adolescents will, however, rely on social media, where there will be no individual to judge the kind of information they search for or the questions they ask. Also, the students stressed the need for more practical examples in our facilities as one of the reasons why they will prefer getting reproductive health information via social media instead of the health facility. On social media, video evidence of questions is provided to illustrate further for students to understand. Considering the age of these students, they would prefer visuals as a means of communication compared to just words or statements.

This aligns with another study examining how teens utilize social media to get reproductive health care. This study identified a barrier to young people using the services provided by adolescent health clinics as the absence of confidentiality at the delivery stations [45]. Facilities have to arrange to give privacy to patients or clients during their sessions, whether via physical boundaries between counseling and professional areas or other appropriate arrangements. Another study in Uganda discovered that most service facilities lacked enclosures to give young girls and boys privacy. Only one higher-order hospital was known to have a site where youth programming might be offered. With this, no healthcare facility had a separate reception area for young people to provide service without interruption from other staff [46].

In addition, many teenagers think it would be humiliating to have their marital status questioned if they were to engage in family planning because most of them will not be married then. Additionally, one person said family planning was not for adolescents but for grownups [44]. In this same survey, A service giver stated his hesitation about delivering contraception to a 13-year-old girl.

Just like every study, this study has certain restrictions. The findings are based on self-reported, individual data that respondents' social desirability may skew due to participants filling out surveys in a school setting.

6. Conclusion

Social media has come to stay. It has started having a tremendous influence on the youth and adolescents who have found it safer and more convenient to consult rather than relying on their parents and families for sexual reproductive information, which in most societies is taboo to discuss. Adolescent heavily rely on social media because there is a lack of access to this information in a safe, friendly and culturally sensitive manner. Those who attempt to obtain this information are either rebuked or tagged as bad. As a result of the stigma associated with getting sexual reproductive health information from peers, family members, and teachers, they find social media the most convenient place to obtain this information. Sex, social media usage, urban or rural residence and adolescent romantic relationships were factors significantly associated with their access to juvenile reproductive health information via social media. Despite the high utilization of social media for reproductive health services, there is no clear-cut policy in Ghana on social media and how to regulate it to ensure that the information put out there is not harmful to the adolescents.

Author details

Rahma Salifu[1] and Abdulai Abubakari[2*]

1 Ghana Health Service, Tamale, Ghana

2 Institute of Interdisciplinary Research (IIR), University for Development Studies, Tamale, Ghana

*Address all correspondence to: abdulai.abubakari@uds.edu.gh

References

[1] Pfeiffer C, Kleeb M, Mbelwa A, Ahorlu C. The use of social media among adolescents in Dar es Salaam and Mtwara, Tanzania. Reproductive Health Matters. 2014;**22**(43):178-186

[2] Kietzmann JH, Hermkens K, McCarthy IP, Silvestre BS. Social media? Get serious! Understanding the functional building blocks of social media. Business Horizons. 2011;**54**(3):241-251

[3] Hightow-weidman LB, Building B, Hill C, Muessig KE, Hill C, Carolina N, et al. Youth. Technology and HIV: Recent Advances and Directions. 2016;**12**(4):500-515

[4] Fung IC, Blankenship EB, Ahweyevu JO, Cooper LK, Duke CH, Carswell SL, et al. Public health implications of image-based social media: A systematic review of instagram, pinterest, tumblr, and flickr. The Permanente Journal. 2020:1-10

[5] Abi-Jaoud E. Smartphones, social media use and youth mental health. Canadian Medical Association Journal. 2020;**192**(6):136-141

[6] Okeleke K. Digital transformation in Tanzania: The role of mobile technology and impact on development goals. GSMA Association. 2019. Available from: www.gsma.com

[7] Olumide AO, Ojengbede OA. The media as a critical determinant of the sexual and reproductive health of adolescents in Ibadan, Nigeria. Sexual and Reproductive Healthcare. 2016;**8**:63-74

[8] Kim B, White K. How can health professionals enhance interpersonal communication with adolescents and young adults to improve health care outcomes?: Systematic literature review. International Journal of Adolescence and Youth. 2018;**3843**:1-21

[9] Akram W, Kumar R. A study on positive and negative effects of social media on society. International Journal of Computer Sciences and Engineering. 2017;**5**(10):347-354

[10] Tripathi M, Singh S, Ghimire S. Effect of social media on human health. Virology & Immunology Journal. 2018;**2**(2):1-10

[11] Choo J, Kang H. Predictors of initial weight loss among women with abdominal obesity: A path model using self-efficacy and health-promoting behaviour. Journal of Advance Nursing. 2014;**71**(5):1087-1097

[12] Litman L, Weinberger-litman S, Goldschein A, Robinson J. Mobile exercise apps and increased leisure time exercise activity: A moderated mediation analysis of the role of self-efficacy and barriers. Journal of Medical Internet Research. 2015;**17**(8):e4142

[13] Anaba EA. Determinants of adolescent sexual and reproductive health service quality in Ghana. American Journal of Preventive Medicine and Public Health. 2020;**6**(1):1-8

[14] Adokiya MN, Cudjoe FK, Yakong VN. Predictors of education and utilization of adolescent-friendly health services among youth in Kumbungu district, Ghana. Journal of Health Research. 2020;**36**(2):311-322

[15] Yussif AS, Lassey A, Ganyaglo GYK, Kantelhardt EJ, Kielstein H. The long-term effects of adolescent pregnancies in a community in Northern Ghana on

subsequent pregnancies and births of the young mothers. Reproductive Health. 2017;**14**(1):1-7

[16] Venkatesh V, Morris M, Davis G, Davis F. User acceptance of information technology: Toward a unified view. MIS Quarterly. 2003;**27**:425-478

[17] Davis FD. Perceived usefulness, perceived ease of use and user acceptance of information technology. MIS Quarterly. 1989;**13**:319-340

[18] Varela FJ, Thompson E, Rosch E. The Embodied Mind: Cognitive Science and Human Experience. 1st ed. Mass: MIT Press, Cambridge; 1991. p. 308

[19] Rogers E. Diffusion of Innovations. 5th ed. Simon and Schuster; 2003. p. 576

[20] Fishbein M, Ajzen I. Belief, Attitude, Intention and Behavior: An Introduction to Theory and Research. 1st ed. Reading: Addison-Wesley Pub. Co.; 1975. p. 578

[21] Davis F, Bagozzi R, Warshaw P. User acceptance of computer technology: A comparison of two theoretical models. Management Science. 1989;**35**:982-1003

[22] Ajzen I. The theory of planned behavior. Organizational Behavior and Human Decision Processes. 1991;**50**:179-211

[23] Compeau DR, Higgins C. Application of social cognitive theory to training for computer skills. Information Systems Research. 1995;**6**:118-143

[24] Taylor S, Todd P. Understanding information technology usage: A test of competing models. Information Systems Research. 1995;**6**:144-176. DOI: 10.1287/isre.6.2.144

[25] Lu J, Yao JE, Chun-Sheng Y. Personal innovativeness, social influence and adoption of wireless internet services via mobile technology. Journal of Strategic Information Systems. 2005;**14**:245-268

[26] Snedecor GW, Cochran WG. Statistical Methods, 8th Edition. Iowa State University Press. 1989. pp. 491

[27] Aranda-Jan CB, Mohutsiwa-Dibe N, Loukanova S. Systematic review on what works, what does not work and why of implementation of mobile health (mHealth) projects in Africa. BMC Public Health. 2014;**14**(1)

[28] Nwalo KIN, Anasi SNI. Access to and use of reproductive health information among in-school adolescent girls in Lagos State, Nigeria. Health Education Journal. 2010;**71**(1):90-101

[29] Plaisime M, Robertson-James C, Mejia L, Núñez A, Wolf J, Reels S. Social media and teens: A needs assessment exploring the potential role of social media in promoting health. Social Media+Society. 2020;**6**(1)

[30] Ihesie CA, Chukwuogo O. Integrating mHealth into adolescent sexual and reproductive health promotion in Nigeria: Prospects and barriers. International Journal of Community Medicine and Public Health. 2017;**4**(11):3931-3941

[31] Gray BJ, Jones AT, Couzens Z, Sagar T, Jones D. University students' behaviours towards accessing sexual health information and treatment. International Journal of STD and AIDS. 2019;**30**(7):671-679

[32] Lim F, Vella SD, Hellard ME. Young people's comfort receiving sexual health information via social media and other sources. 2014, International Journal of STD & AIDS. 2014;**25**(14):1003-1008

[33] Goodyear V, Kathleen Armour HW. The Impact of Social Media on Young

People's Health and Wellbeing: Evidence, Guidelines and Actions. University of Birmingham; 2018

[34] Duggan M, Aaron SR, Lee Perrin A, Porteus M, Page D, Shannon GS. Mobile messaging and Social Media -2015. Pew Research Center 2015. Available from: http://www.pewinternet.org/2015/08/19/mobile-messaging-and-social-media-2015/

[35] Wendy N, Santosh K, Albert S, Carrie V, Tisha W, William T, et al. Advancing the Science of mHealth. Journal of Health Communication. 2012;**17**:sup1:5-10. DOI: 10.1080/10810730.2012.677394

[36] Rokicki S. Assessing the reach and effectiveness of mHealth: Evidence from a reproductive health program for adolescent girls in Ghana. BMC Public Health. 2017;**17**(969):1-14

[37] Ippoliti NB, Engle KL. Meet us on the phone: Mobile phone programs for adolescent sexual and reproductive health in low-to-middle income countries. Reproductive Health. 2017;**1-8**. DOI: 10.1186/s12978-016-0276-z

[38] Hampshire K, Porter G, Asiedu S, Mariwah S, Abane A, Robson E, et al. Social science & medicine informal m-health: How are young people using mobile phones to bridge healthcare gaps in Sub-Saharan Africa? Social Science & Medicine. 2015;**142**:90-99

[39] Chib A, Velthoven M, Van & Car J. mHealth adoption in low-resource environments: A review of the use of mobile healthcare in developing countries. Journal of Health Communication. 2014;**0**:1-31

[40] Blumenstock JE, Hall MG, Eagle N. Divided We Call: Disparities in access and use of mobile phones in Rwanda. Information Technologies International Development. 2012;**8**(2):1-16

[41] Asare BYA, Aryee SE, Kotoh AM. Sexual behaviour and the utilization of youth friendly health Services: A cross-sectional study among urban youth in Ghana. International Journal of Africa Nursing Sciences. 2020;**13**

[42] Sudhakar BP, Shrivastava SR. A cross sectional study of knowledge and practices about reproductive health among female adolescents in an urban slum of Mumbai. Journal of Family and Reproductive Health. 2011;**5**(4):119-126

[43] Ilori OR, Awodutire PO, Ilori OS. Awareness and utilization of adolescent reproductive health services among in-school adolescents in urban and rural communities in Oyo State. Nigerian Medical Journal: Journal of the Nigeria Medical Association. 2020;**61**(2):67

[44] Motuma A, Syre T, Egata G, Kenay A. Utilization of youth friendly services and associated factors among youth in Harar town, east Ethiopia: A mixed method study. BMC Health Services Research. 2016:1-10

[45] Binu W, Marama T, Gerbaba M, Sinaga M. Sexual and reproductive health services utilization and associated factors among secondary school students in Nekemte town, Ethiopia. Reproductive Health. 2018;**15**:64

[46] Bukenya JN, Mulogo E, Kibira SPS, Muhumuza C, Atuyambe LM. HHS public access. Annals of Global Health. 2017;**2**(3)

Section 2

Hormonal Contraceptions Methods

Chapter 3

Family Planning

Anna Maria Paoletti, Gian Benedetto Melis, Bruno Piras, Monica Pilloni, Pierina Zedda, Maria Francesca Marotto, Valerio Vallerino, Anna Melis, Valeria Taccori, Virginia Melis, Giulia Melis, Elena Giancane and Manuela Neri

Abstract

The contraception (the term is the fusion between "contra", against, and conception): includes all methods that prevent conception. According to the physiology of human reproduction, the contraceptive methods can prevent the fecundation by hindering the female and male gametes meeting. In these mechanisms we include: The abstinence by sexual intercourse around the ovulatory phase of the cycle; The use of barriers that block contact between male gametes and female genitalia; The use of methods impeding the ascent of spermatozoa through the female genital tracts (intrauterine devices). The prevention of the oocyte from being available (hormonal contraceptives or oral contraceptives, OC). In this category there is the availability of short acting reversible contraception (SARC) (pill, vaginal ring, patch), and the long acting reversible contraception (LARC) (progestin implants). The ideal contraceptive method has to respond to four fundamental principles: efficacy, safety, reversibility, tolerability. The authors will discuss all the above contraceptive methods with the evaluation of indications and contraindications to each method.

Keywords: hormonal contraceptives, short acting reversible contraception (SARC), long acting reversible contraception (LARC), intrauterine devices, male and female condom

1. Introduction

The family planning identifies the mechanisms through which a couple organizes the time for the conception and in many cases, especially for economic reasons, it is necessary to avoid the pregnancy for a short or long time. The contraception (the term is the fusion between "contra", against, and conception): includes all methods that prevent conception. The history of humanity is marked by the search for contraceptive methods that have found an important milestone in the development of strategies that hinder the meeting of male and female gametes (condom, hood, diaphragm). However, the preferred contraceptive method has become the one that prevent the availability of the female gamete, because in this way the couple has the advantage to plan conception at the most suitable time, without giving up sexuality. According to the physiology of human reproduction, the contraceptive methods can prevent the fecundation by hindering the female and male gametes meeting. In these mechanisms we include:

- The abstinence by sexual intercourse around the ovulatory phase of the cycle;
- The use of barriers that block contact between male gametes and female genitalia;
- The use of methods impeding the ascent of spermatozoa through the female genital tracts (intrauterine devices or IUD);
- The prevention of the oocyte from being available (hormonal contraceptives or oral contraceptives, OC). In this category there is the availability of short acting reversible contraception (SARC) (pill, vaginal ring, patch), and the long acting reversible contraception (LARC) (progestin implants).

The ideal contraceptive method has to respond to four fundamental principles: efficacy, safety, reversibility, tolerability.

2. The abstinence by sexual intercourse around the ovulatory phase of the cycle

For this method it is necessary to identify the time period of the ovulation through the following mechanisms: a. the calendar method that identifies ovulation basing on the interval between one menstruation and the next, considering the post-ovulatory phase lasting 14 days; b. the evaluation of cervical mucus, abundant and racy in the ovulatory period and with increased thickness in the postovulatory period; c. the assessment of the basal temperature, which increases during the luteal phase (after the ovulation) in relationship to the increase of progesterone secretion and has a reduction near the ovulatory phase; d. the identification of the ovulatory LH peak through monoclonal antibodies capable of binding LH molecules in the urine. All these methods do not interfere on the safety and on reversibility, but they are characterized by both a bad tolerability and efficacy [1]. With a perfect (but very difficult) use of these methods, the contraceptive efficacy is included in a range between 0.4–5% of unwanted pregnancies within a year of use [2].

3. The use of barriers that block contact between male gametes and female genitalia

3.1 The male condom

The male condom is a popular and known method of contraception. However, not everyone knows the differences in their composition. Latex condom protects against unwanted pregnancy and sexually transmitted diseases (STDs), including HIV and Herpes virus, when used correctly [3]. Other materials used in the male condom are polyisoprene, polyurethane and the material derived from the intestine of lamb. Faced with a low risk of slipping and breaking, due to its high elasticity, the polyisoprene-based condom is burdened by poor sensitivity between the partners [4]. The one based on polyurethane is the thinnest and while ensuring high sensitivity because it is thinner than the same latex condom, it is burdened by the risk of slipping and breaking [5]. The condom obtained from the intestine of lamb does not protect against STDs [6]. The contraceptive efficacy of this method, calculated as percent of unwanted pregnancies within a year of use is 18% for typical use and 2% for perfect use [2].

3.2 The female condom

The female condom is less used and known than the male one. It consists of a thin latex sheath that adapts to the vagina. In practice, the closed part with a ring is inserted into the vagina, while the open part, with another ring, remains outside the vagina. It can be inserted 8 hours before the intercourse. It protects against STDs, but its insertion is difficult and, moreover, it can be disadvantageous in sexual intercourse for both partners [7]. The contraceptive efficacy of this method, calculated as percent of unwanted pregnancies within a year of use is 21% for typical use and 5% for perfect use [2].

3.3 The vaginal diaphragm

The diaphragm is a kind of cup-shaped lid, made of latex or silicone. Its placement in the vagina is facilitated by a flexible structure at the edges of the diaphragm. It should be positioned to cover the cervix entirely. Its size should be evaluated by a gynecologist based on the size of each individual woman's cervix [8]. It is used in combination with a spermicide, so it offers a greater contraceptive treatment than the male condom alone. After intercourse, it must remain in place for at least 6 hours, but no longer than 24 hours [8]. The positioning period correlates with the risk of urinary infections and urinary stagnation. After careful hygiene, it can be used for more intercourses as opposed to male and female condoms [8]. The contraceptive efficacy of this method, calculated as percent of unwanted pregnancies within a year of use is 12% for typical use and 6% for perfect use [2].

3.4 The cervical cap

The cervical cap is dome-shaped and is made of silicone. It adapts to the cervix, held in place by the vaginal walls [9]. Thanks to a cord it is possible to easily remove it. Like the diaphragm, it must be used with spermicides. Also inserted 42 hours before sexual intercourse, it should not be removed before six hours after sexual intercourse, but no later than 24 hours [9]. Compared to the diaphragm it has a lower risk of urinary infections, but it is contraindicated in women with neoplastic or preneoplastic pathologies of the uterine cervix. It is not suitable for subjects with anatomical anomalies of the uterine cervix [9]. The contraceptive efficacy of this method, calculated as percent of unwanted pregnancies within a year of use is 24% for typical use and 20% for perfect use, in pluriparous women, whereas it is better in nulliparous women (12% for typical use, 9% for perfect use) [2].

3.5 The spermicides

The spermicides are substances based on nonoxynol-9. The mechanism through which they exert the contraception is the destruction of spermatozoa. They are available in different forms: gel, cream, vaginal film, sponges. They have to be applied at least 15 hours before the sexual intercourse. Irritation on both the vagina and the penis are often reported [10]. The efficacy in reducing the risk of STDs has recently been discussed with not encouraging results [11]. The contraceptive efficacy of this method, calculated as percent of unwanted pregnancies within a year of use is 28% for typical use and 18% for perfect use [2].

4. The use of methods impeding the ascent of spermatozoa through the female genital tracts

Intrauterine devices (IUDs) are defined LARC in relationship to the long-lasting contraceptive effect (years), thus they have the advantage of the absence of daily intake of OC. The contraindications to their use are very few. Although poorly used in Europe (10% of women using contraception), IUDs have widespread use in Asia (40% of women). Compared to copper IUDs (Cu-IUDs), which act by exerting a spermicidal effect [12, 13], levonorgestrel-intrauterine system (LNG-IUS) prevents sperm passing through the uterine cervix because it thickens the cervical mucus [12]. Unlike the Cu-IUD, LNG-IUS does not increase the number of endometrial leukocytes, and exerts a suppressive effect on the endometrium, decreasing its thickness in relation to local LNG release [13]. This mechanism of LNG-IUS has been reported to be favorable to reducing menstrual flow and dysmenorrhea [14, 15], whereas in Cu-IUD users increased menstrual flow and dysmenorrhea have been reported [16]. The first LNG-IUS is a 32x32 mm T-shaped device, containing a reserve of 52 mg of LNG (release of approximately 18 mcg/day), approved for a duration of action of 5 years [17]. Due to its size, it is intended for use in women who have already given birth, with a cervical canal compliant with introduction. The need to have a similar contraceptive to offer to the adolescents and the nulliparous women has led to the development of a smaller IUS (30x28 mm) and with LNG content of only 13.5 mg, which induces a very reduced passage of the hormone in the bloodstream (approximately 160 pg./mL in the first 7 days after placement, reduced to up to 60 pg./mL after 3 years), with fewer systemic side effects than the previous one. The applicator (diameter of 3.8 mm compared to 4.75 mm of the previous one) also favors use in adolescents and nulliparous [18–20]. The contraceptive duration is 3 years. Recently, an IUS of the same size has been proposed, but with a higher content of LNG (19.5 mg), so as to allow the contraceptive effect for 5 years [21]. There are very few contraindications to LNG-IUDs [22]. Among these: the presence of antiphospholipid antibodies; the history of breast cancer [22]. In these cases, it is possible to opt for a Cu-IUD [22], or an irreversible contraception, such as female or male sterilization. The contraceptive efficacy of Cu-IUD, calculated as percent of unwanted pregnancies within a year of use is 0.8% for typical use and 0.2% for perfect use [2]. The contraceptive efficacy of LNG-IUS, calculated as percent of unwanted pregnancies within a year of use is 0.2% for typical use and 0.2% for perfect use [2].

5. The prevention of the oocyte from being available (hormonal contraceptives or oral contraceptives, OC). It includes also vaginal ring, and patches as SARC and progestin implant as LARC

5.1 Introduction

In modern society, in which the self-determination of the individual and free will have acquired central importance, the possibility of an effective contraception has been a great achievement for women. In fact, making effective contraception means being able to freely choose when to plan the pregnancy and the creation of a family and, consequently, allow the woman to dedicate her time to what she deems most appropriate for her life and her own growth. It is not a coincidence that, starting from the 1970s, when OC began to spread especially in the United States, the prevalence of women with degrees in various disciplines had a peak of growth [23]. Studies of economics applied to medicine illustrate how the adoption of birth control improves economic growth in developing countries, because with fewer dependent children and the ability to plan pregnancy, women can participate more actively to the workforce and increase the productivity of the country [24]. Moreover, the family planning, implemented thanks to effective contraception, can also lead to other demonstrated social benefits, such as an improvement in maternal BMI (body mass index) (linked to a greater temporal distance between one pregnancy and the next), a reduction of the infant mortality, a higher level of child education and schooling, as well as a better overall health status of offspring [24].

It has been estimated that in developing countries the use of OC has led to a reduction in maternal mortality by up to 40%, thanks to the prevention of unwanted pregnancies that would result in clandestine or unsafe abortions, and avoiding pregnancy in high-risk or multiparous women, penalized by higher mortality [25].

Finally, adolescents are among the categories most at risk of unwanted pregnancy and among those most at risk of adverse outcomes if the pregnancy is continued, such as premature birth, low fetal birth weight, greater morbidity and neonatal mortality [26]. Nonetheless, adolescent pregnancy, as well as the use of voluntary abortion, can have significant psychological consequences in young women, with a greater risk of mood disorders in subsequent years [27].

In fact, the advent of OC can be considered a great achievement not only for the affirmation of woman's autonomy, but also for the approval of the whole society.

5.2 History of contraception and evolution of contraceptives

In the history, the first evidence of an attempt at contraception dates back to ancient Egypt, where some papyri describe the use of natural products, such as honey or acacia leaves, to be inserted into the vagina close to intercourse. Ancient Greco-Roman sources speak of herbal products that could cause sterility or induce abortion. Several descriptions of rudimentary condoms appear in history, among which the lambskin condom proposed by Casanova in the eighteenth century as a method of preventing pregnancy and sexually transmitted diseases is certainly characteristic [28]. However, only in the twentieth century was there a turning point in contraception, both for the spread of the need for birth control in the population and for the discovery of effective contraceptive methods.

Faced with a strong social need, Margaret Sanger, an American nurse and writer, pioneer of reproductive and women's rights, opened the first clinic for family planning in Brooklyn in 1916. Shortly after, in 1921, the British scientist Marie Stopes founded one in the UK [28]. But advances in medical science made their contribution to contraception only in the mid-twentieth century, when the first molecules with progestin activity were synthesized, thanks to the work of scientists such as G. Pincus, M.C. Chang and J. Rock, who led to the discovery that these molecules were capable of inhibiting ovulation. Thus, the FDA approved Enovid in 1957, a combination of synthetic estrogen-progestins (mestranol 150 mcg and noretinodrel 9.5 mg), first as a therapy for the control of menstrual disorders, and then, in 1960, as a contraceptive method [29]. In Italy, only in 1971 the contraceptive "pill" was accepted by a sentence of the Constitutional Court as a method of birth control.

Since the invention of the first contraceptive pill, in just over 60 years, advances in pharmacology have now led to numerous OC solutions, with different formulations, methods of administration, short and long-term duration of action, as well as different active molecules, which adapt to the multiple needs and preferences of the female audience. As said previously, the ideal characteristics of a contraceptive method are: its effectiveness, that is the ability to achieve the goal of preventing pregnancy; its reversibility, or the remission of the effect after the suspension of the method; the safety for health and tolerability, because a product that improves a woman's quality of life cannot cause damage to health or cause side effects or discomfort in the intake, which would affect its use. Considering this premise, in the evolution of OC, on the one hand there have been progress in the name of safety, while guaranteeing contraceptive efficacy, characterized by a reduction in the dosage of the estrogenic component (the synthetic estrogen ethinyl estradiol, EE) and from the discovery of new progestogen molecules that have a better metabolic and pharmacodynamic profile on steroid hormone receptors. On the other hand, the same has been done to improve the acceptance by the woman of the contraceptive method, and therefore the tolerability itself, with the creation of different regimens of administration in addition to the oral one (transdermal, transvaginal, subcutaneous, intrauterine), short or long acting [28].

The main health risk in Ref. to OC is that of thromboembolic events, especially venous thromboembolic events (VTE) and secondarily arterial thromboembolic events (ATE), since estrogens have a general effect of hyper-coagulability. In fact, they increase the synthesis in the liver and the biological activity of pro-coagulant proteins such as fibrinogen, prothrombin and other coagulation factors, while reducing the synthesis and activity of anticoagulant factors such as the S protein [30]. The OC, therefore, has always been associated with an increased risk of VTE, which varies according to the dose of estrogen and the associated progestogen. It is very conditioned by additional individual risk factors such as age, weight, the habit smoking and other condition, such as migraine with aura [31]. The reduction of the EE dosage in OC, from more than 50 mcg used in the old OC combinations to the currently used doses of 15–30 mcg, has allowed to reduce the thromboembolic risk by about half, but without completely eliminating it [32]. The associated progestin compound is capable of modulating the overall biological estrogenic effect of the OC and the effect on the blood coagulation, in relationship to its ability to act also on other steroid receptors, such as androgen receptors [33, 34].

One of the most important recent population studies, which assessed the thromboembolic risk associated with the use of OCs over 10 years of observation, reported an absolute risk of VTE in women not using OC of 3 cases out of 10.000/year; the risk increases to 6.3 cases per 10.000/year in women using OC. It decreases after the first year of use; but with the same EE dose and length of use, the compounds that have the lowest risk profile are those containing LNG as progestin, compared to the other OC with progestin such as desogestrel (DSG), gestodene (GSD), drospirenone (DRSP) and cyproterone acetate (CPA), which demonstrated a higher relative risk than the EE/LNG combination [32]. For this reason, to date, the OC with EE + LNG is the one considered as the referent in clinical studies that evaluate the thromboembolic risk associated with OC. In any case, it must be considered that the risk of VTE events associated with pregnancy is higher, equal to 17 cases out of 10.000 pregnancies [35].

The progestin component is the one that has undergone major changes in the evolution of OC (**Table 1**). Thanks to the action on the progesterone receptors at a central level, the progestin compound guarantees the inhibition of ovulation and the contraceptive effect. On the other hand, the ability of the progestin to bind and activate other receptors for steroid hormones, such as those for androgens, glucocorticoids and mineralocorticoids, affects the metabolic safety profile and the appearance of unpleasant side effects [34].

The first progestogen molecules used in OC were testosterone derivatives, which maintained the androgenic activity and could cause manifestations such as acne, seborrhea and hirsutism and, mainly, negative effects on glucidic and insulin metabolisms. Advances in pharmacology have subsequently created compounds with greater selectivity and potency on progesterone receptors and more similar to progesterone itself. Thus, modern progestin compounds used in OC, such as DRSP or dienogest (DNG), are characterized by this selectivity, plus the absence of activation of glucocorticoid and androgen receptors, but rather a mild antiandrogenic activity, which may be clinically useful for managing some symptoms complained of by women [34, 36].

Progestinic compounds	AE	EST	AND	AA	GLU	AM
Progesterone	+	—	—	+/−	+	+
Chlormadinone acetate	+	—	—	+	+	—
Ciproterone acetate	+	—	—	+++	+	—
Dienogest	+	—	—	++	—	—
Drospirenone	+	—	—	+	—	+
Desogestrel/Etonorgestrel	+	—	+	—	+/−	—
Gestodene	+	—	+	—	+/−	+
Levonorgestrel	+	—	+	—	—	—
Medrossiprogesterone acetate	+	—	+/−	—	+	—
Nomegestrolo acetate	+	—	—	+	—	—
Noretisterone	+	+	+	—	—	—
Norelgestromin	+	—	+	—	—	—

AE: antiestrogenic, EST: estrogenic, AND: androgenic, AA: antiandrogenic, GLU: glucocorticoid, AM: antimineralcorticoid.

Table 1.
Biological activities of progestinic compounds.

5.2.1 Contraception with "natural estrogen"

EE has remained a pillar in the OC for about 50 years, although the doses used have been progressively reduced. The use for contraception of an estrogen molecule analogous to 17β estradiol (E2) synthesized by the human body has always been limited by the lower power of E2 compared to EE on estrogen receptors and, consequently, by the inability to stabilize the endometrium and subsequent bleeding [37]. Only after the discovery of progestin compounds with a high power on progesterone receptors and a high antiproliferative activity on the endometrium, it was possible to create an OC with E2, which would allow good control of uterine bleeding. The potential metabolic advantages of using E2 in place of EE are many: the lower activation of estrogen receptors in the liver results in a lower stimulation of the synthesis of multiple proteins, including those involved in the mechanisms of coagulation, the sex hormone binding globulin (SHBG), angiotensinogen, or some lipoproteins [38].

The lower influence on the renin-angiotensin-aldosterone system (RAAS) determines a lower influence of E2 on blood pressure, the slight increase of which is a possible side effect of EE-based OCs, due to a mild sodium-retentive effect. The clinical evidence, in this regard, does not report a modification of the blood pressure values measured during treatment with OC based on E2 [39, 40]. Furthermore, in the evaluation of cardiovascular risk associated with OC, many studies have evaluated the dosage of coagulation markers (fibrinogen, D-dimer, protein S), of lipoproteins and triglycerides, of glucose metabolism, and their modifications during OC treatment. Despite being a laboratory-only evaluation, E2-based OCs induce only minimal or no modification of these parameters, with effects that in some cases have been shown to be significantly better than OCs with EE/LNG [33, 41, 42]. In light of these data, in theory, OCs containing E2 should have a better cardio-vascular and metabolic safety profile. However, the evidence comes mainly from studies evaluating lower cardio-metabolic outcomes (blood pressure, laboratory values) and not the effects of real clinical interest such as VTE or ATE. The young age of E2 OCs, compared to more than 60 years of experience with EE, requires time to evaluate the real impact of this promising new contraception with large-scale surveillance studies.

The only "real life" population study, carried out on routine clinical practice, which investigated the safety profile from the cardiovascular point of view of OCs containing E2 valerate (EV) (specifically the first commercialized combination of EV/DNG), is the INAS-SCORE study (The International Active Surveillance study "Safety of Contraceptives: Role of Estrogens"), published in 2016 [43]. As a prospective, non-interventional cohort study, conducted in the USA and in 7 different European countries, the INAS-SCORE study recruited more than 50.000 women with a new OC prescription, following them for a follow-up period of 2 to 5 and a half years, for a total of more than 100.000 women per year observation. The main objective of the study was to evaluate the incidence of venous and arterial thromboembolic events occurring in women with a new EV/DNG prescription compared to "other" OCs and, in particular, to the EE/LNG subgroup. From the first analysis of the study results, there is a risk of VTE of 7.2 new cases per 10.000 women/year (95% CI: 3.3–13.7) with EV/DNG, 9.1 per 10.000 women/year (95% CI: 6.9–11.8) with other OCs, 9.9 of 10.000 women/year (95% CI: 4.8–18.3) with EE/LNG and 3.5 of 10.000 women/year (95% CI: 1.6–6.7) in the population of women not using OCs. Similarly, the incidence of ATE was also lower in the group of EV/DNG users. The relative risk of VTE with the EE/LNG OC was not higher than that of the other OCs or the EE/LNG combination, while the analysis of European data (where the use of EV/DNG was more widespread) revealed a significantly lower risk of VTE of EV/DNG compared to the class including all other OCs. The INAS-SCORE study, despite being a single first evidence, therefore demonstrated with high statistical strength that contraception with EV/DNG is associated with a cardiovascular risk similar, if not even lower, to the EE/LNG combination and the other COCs [43]. The extension phase of INAS-SCORE study focused on VTE and ATE with an implementation of follow-up procedures. More than 50.000 OC users were followed for 2 to 7 years. In the Europe database the results show that the EV/DNG exerts a lower risk of VTE and ATE vs. all OCs with a similar or lower risk vs. EE/LNG [44].

There are two contraceptive formulations containing E2 currently on the market: the combination of E2V and DNG (E2/DNG) (Qlaira®, Bayer S.p.A.), multiphasic OC with dynamic dosage with 26 active tablets plus 2 placebo, approved in Italy since 2009 [45] (Klaira®, Bayer S.p.A.), and the association of micronized E2 with nomegestrol acetate (NOMAC) (Zoely®, Theramex), in a monophasic regimen with a dosage of 1.5 mg and 2.5 mg respectively and with a 24 + 4 administration schedule (24 active tablets plus 4 placebo), available on the market since 2011 [46].

E2V represents the esterified form of E2 which allows for a greater bioavailability of estrogen when administered orally; 1 mg of E2V is equivalent to 0.76 mg of E2. After being absorbed, E2V is split in the liver into E2 and valeric acid [47]. The DNG associated in OC with E2V is a derivative of 19-nortestosterone with a peculiar chemical structure as it is the only progestin compound to associate properties of both 19-nortestosterone derivatives and progesterone derivatives, which leads to an high action on progesterone receptors and antiandrogenic activity, equal to 40% compared to that of CPA (the progestin compound with greater antiandrogenic activity [48]). The anti-estrogenic action of DNG at the uterine level is protective for the endometrium by stabilizing bleeding, and contributes to the contraceptive efficacy due to the effect on cervical mucus [37, 49]. Contraceptive treatment with E2V/DNG was associated with an improvement in the lipid profile, with a decrease in LDL cholesterol levels and an increase in HDL cholesterol, and with a lesser influence on carbohydrate metabolism parameters and clotting markers, compared to the combination EE/LNG [34, 41, 50].

The second contraceptive with natural estrogen associates E2 with NOMAC, a derivative of 19nor-progesterone with powerful progestin activity more marked than that of natural progesterone, anti-estrogenic activity and mild antiandrogenic activity. Having no androgenic, glucocorticoid or mineralocorticoid activity, NOMAC has proved to be a safe progestin from a cardiovascular and metabolic point of view [51]. Studies reported so far show that E2/NOMAC does not modify the lipidic and glucose metabolism, does not induce significant changes in blood pressure and C-reactive protein and has an almost negligible influence on the blood coagulation system [42, 52]. During treatment, no changes in bone metabolism and bone mineral density were observed [53].

5.2.2 Prospects for the future of OC with natural estrogen

Although the introduction of natural estrogen in OC has created a great alternative to traditional compounds with EE, it is not surprising that pharmacological research is still active in seeking and combining new molecules, always in the name of a better profile of safety and acceptability of the drug. One of the molecules that is most arousing curiosity for a possible future use both in OC and in hormone replacement therapy for menopause is estetrol (E4). Estetrol is also a "natural" hormone, since it is synthesized by the fetal liver during pregnancy. Although known for a long time and considered a weak estrogen, E4 has aroused low interest until the discovery of a poor pharmacokinetic and pharmacodynamic interaction in the liver [54]. In vitro and in vivo studies have shown that E4 does not induce hepatic synthesis of SHBG and does not affect the activity of cytochrome P450, which inhibits ovulation in a dose-dependent manner and which acts as estrogen in the vagina, uterus and bone [55]. These premises have supported phase II studies with the use of E4 as an OC in combination with DRSP or LNG, which have shown efficacy in inhibiting ovulation, with a low metabolic impact on the synthesis of liver proteins [56–58]; phase III studies show the efficacy and safety of the OC containing 15 mg of E4+3 mg of DRSP [59].

5.3 Different way of estroprogestin OC

To reduce the discomfort of taking the pill daily, different routes of administration have been available. These include the transdermal route of administration with the patch containing EE and the progestin norelgestromin. The patch, applied to the abdomen, arm or shoulder, ensures the disposal of contraceptive doses for one week. Therefore, it must be replaced weekly. Another route of administration is the vaginal one. The vaginal ring releases daily a very low dose of EE and the progestin etonorgestrel (ETN). Both of these routes of administration have the advantage of ensuring constant doses of hormones and are not conditioned by intestinal absorption. This is very beneficial for women with food intolerances. Furthermore, with these routes of administration an excellent cycle control was found, as well as an excellent metabolic profile on the lipid and glucose side [60, 61].

5.4 Hormonal contraception with progestogen only compound

In many cases where the use of estrogen (including E2) is contraindicated, progestogen compound alone can be used [22]. The oral formulation contains 75mcg of DSG. This pill must be taken every day and the most annoying side effect is the irregular bleeding. The progestin, especially ETN, can also be used as a LARC. The ETN implant releases enough hormone for its contraceptive effect for at least three years. Even with the implantation of ETN the most notable side effect is irregular bleeding [62]. The absence of other serious side effects and its wide spectrum of application make the contraceptive with progestin only in both SARC and LARC formulations an excellent choice for effective, safe and reversible contraception.

Recently, a SARC with the only progestin compound, contained DRSP at the daily dose of 4 mg in a formulation of 24 active pills plus 4 placebo pills, was proposed with the aim to reduce the irregular bleeding in comparison with the only DSG. This contraceptive method demonstrated an excellent efficacy [63, 64] associated with a good tolerability in relationship to a minor irregular bleeding in comparison with DSG only pill [65].

5.5 Non-contraceptive benefits of hormonal contraception

Although the therapeutic goal of OC is the prevention of conception and pregnancy, it can confer multiple additional health and quality of life benefits to women, which are often little known to the female public. Under this point of view, contraception can be used with a "therapeutic" goal. The extra-contraceptive benefits can derive directly from the contraceptive mechanism of action (the inhibition of the ovulation), or they can depend on a direct action of the hormonal components. Most of the additional benefits are obtained on the symptoms that often occur during menstrual cyclicality, such as dysmenorrhea, menstrual headache, premenstrual symptoms, peri-ovulatory pain and ovarian cyst formation, heavy menstrual bleeding and symptoms of hyperandrogenism. Other no less important benefits include the prevention of ectopic pregnancies, pelvic inflammatory disease, oncological risk (reduction of ovarian, endometrial and colorectal cancer), and the improvement of endometriosis symptoms [66, 67]. The set of benefits that can be obtained from long-lasting contraception in women without contraindications thus creates an absolutely favorable benefit/risk ratio (**Figure 1**).

The direct anti-ovulatory and endometrial effect of OC is capable of effectively treating dysmenorrhea and heavy menstrual bleeding. Dysmenorrhea, especially primary dysmenorrhea, is believed to be linked to an increased production or individual susceptibility to the effect of prostaglandins: the premenstrual hormonal fall, in particular of progesterone, favors an increase in the synthesis of prostaglandins at the endometrial level [68], therefore, abolition of ovulation with OC, counteracts the etiopathogenetic mechanisms of dysmenorrhea. Furthermore, OCs lead to a lower stimulation of endometrial proliferation, with consequent reduction of menstrual fluid and the levels of prostaglandins produced during menstruation, therefore of the uterine contractions necessary to allow menstrual flow [69]. Thanks to these actions, it is well established that different types and different formulations of contraceptives are effective remedies for dysmenorrhea [69]. Even the newest OC with a low dose of EE or containing E2 have shown good results in the control of dysmenorrhea [39, 70, 71], DNG is effective in relieving dysmenorrhea as it has an additional inhibitory action at the level of cyclooxygenase-2 m-RNA, demonstrated by in vitro studies, which allows to reduce the synthesis of prostaglandins [72]. With regard to heavy menstrual cycles, one of the most frequent causes of anemia in women, since they often result from an imbalance in the synthesis of progesterone, when taking an

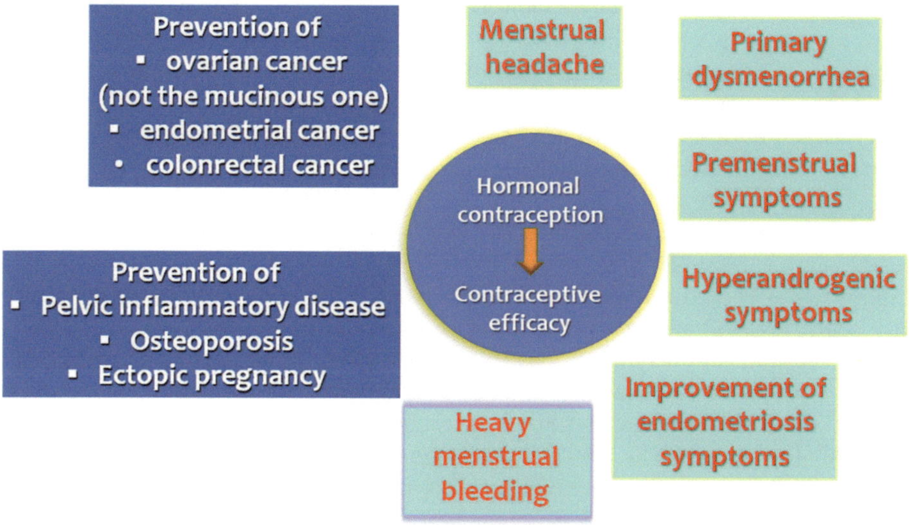

Figure 1.
The contraceptive efficacy of hormonal contraception is associated with many beneficial effects on woman's symptoms dependent on cyclical changes of sexual steroids and on the inhibition of ovulation.

OC an antiproliferative effect on the endometrium is obtained, which have the ability to improve this deleterious menstrual symptom [73]. The new contraceptives with natural estrogen seem even more effective than those with EE in reducing menstrual bleeding, as demonstrated by a comparative study between an OC with E2V/DNG compared with a compound of EE/LNG [74]. In fact, the dynamic multiphase regimen of the E2V/DNG mimics the physiological modifications of the woman's menstrual cycle, with a predominance of estrogen which guarantees endometrial proliferation during the first part of the cycle, and a dominance of DNG in the advanced phase that ensures the maturation and stability of the endometrium; the short 2-day hormone-free interval is sufficient to guarantee the appearance of withdrawal bleeding, which is mostly scarce or sometimes absent [75]. Furthermore, maintaining a stable plasma concentration of hormones has shown an improvement in other symptoms related to the menstrual cycle, such as the menstrual headache [76].

Among the other cyclical disorders that can benefit from an OC is premenstrual syndrome (PMS) or simply the set of unpleasant symptoms such as irritability, decreased mood, headache, tension and swelling, which often anticipate the menstruation. PMS can affect up to 30–40% of women of reproductive age [77], most often with mild symptoms, but in some cases the manifestations may involve considerable discomfort. The etiopathogenesis of PMS is currently unknown, but ovarian steroids, their cyclic fluctuation and their action both on neurotransmitters and neurosteroids in the central nervous system are likely to have a causal action [78]. An interesting epidemiological survey conducted in England on 974 women aged between 20 and 34 years (PMS found in 24% of these) showed a significantly lower prevalence of PMS symptoms in users of OCs, regardless of the type of contraceptive [79]. Both the use of extended intake regimens compared to cyclic ones [80], and some estrogen-progestogen combinations, have shown greater efficacy in the control of this symptomatology: in particular the OC with EE/DRSP, likely in relationship to the antimineralcorticoid and central activity of the DRSP. This OC reduces the premenstrual manifestations compared to the OC with EE/LNG [81] a remarkable result was also observed with the combination E2/NOMAC [82], probably due to a direct central effect of this progestogen. DNG could also have beneficial effects on mood or cognitive functions for an action at the level of the central nervous system. For example, in the context of menopausal hormone replacement therapy it has been reported that treatment with E2 and DNG has achieved an improvement in alertness and cognitive functions better to E2 therapy alone, with a documented activation of some brain areas on electroencephalography [83].

5.6 Tolerability of the contraceptive and therapeutic adherence

The tolerability of the OC is one of the most relevant aspects because it is what mainly conditions adherence to treatment and its continuity over time. If the contraceptive method is poorly tolerated, it will be suspended or used discontinuously, and the direct consequence is the loss of contraceptive efficacy and the uselessness of the method itself. On the other hand, tolerability and adherence to treatment are certainly improved if the contraceptive confers benefits on the general quality of life, and if the woman is aware of the safety of the drug she is taking and of the risk/benefit ratio. Despite all the progress that has been witnessed in the creation of increasingly safer contraceptives that are well suited to the various preferences that every woman may have, the analysis of the 2016 ISTAT data highlights that the use of OC so-called short-acting in Italy it is less than 15%. But in addition to the low use of effective contraceptives found in the population of Italian women, another negative fact to be noted is that a detected number of women who start a OC use stop it within a year of therapy. An interesting interview conducted through online questionnaires on more than 5000 women users of OC, in various European countries, America, Russia and Australia, highlighted in all countries a high rate of interruption of the treatment; the main reason for the interruption-change of the reported contraceptive is the appearance of side effects, which vary from 25 to 60% between countries [84]. In Italy, the survey found a contraceptive treatment interruption rate of 44% [84]. Even considering the most recent OCs with low doses of EE and II-III generation progestin compound, which are expected to show an higher tolerability profile, another Italian survey reported a high discontinuation rate, around 35%, with 25% of women who stop for the onset of adverse effects, in particular, in order of frequency: bleeding irregularities, weight gain, water retention, headache, gastrointestinal symptoms, mood changes, androgenic symptoms, decreased libido, breast tenderness [85].

More generally, population studies that analyze the problem of therapeutic continuity with various contraceptive methods, show a continuation with OCs at 12 months, which varies according to the case series from 55 to 70% approximately [2, 86]. The problem is particularly relevant in adolescents and young women, where an unwanted pregnancy is associated with greater risks for health, for the outcome of the pregnancy itself and for psychological well-being. An interesting survey conducted on a sample of almost 7500 women in Washington state, aimed to compare adherence at 12 months with different methods of contraception divided into SARC (oral OC, vaginal ring, transdermal patch and contraception with progestin only) and LARC (intrauterine contraception, subcutaneous implant of progestin compound), precisely in the various age groups: given that the adolescent age, between 14 and 19 years, showed the most low percentages of continuity at 12 months, this was in any case higher than 80% with the LARC, while with the SARC it was lower, by 44% in the youngest and by 52% from 20 years of age: more than 50% of women who used SARC were not satisfied with the treatment [87]. For this reason, considering both the greater efficacy in the context of everyday life, and the highest adherence, the American guidelines recommend LARC as the first contraceptive choice in adolescents [88]. Certainly, a low profile of adverse events and good bleeding control, improving the tolerability of the contraceptive, can also improve compliance with OCs. Another discomfort that is sometimes complained of while taking OC concerns libido and the sexual sphere. In the light of the pharmacodynamic characteristics of E2 compared to EE and of the two associated progestogens DNG and NOMAC, which are devoid of androgenic and glucocorticoid activity, contraception with natural estrogen pills it would expect metabolic neutrality (and therefore on body weight) and a scarce influence on the mechanisms underlying salt and water retention. If we consider that weight gain, swelling and water retention are among the side effects of OC most reported and most feared by the female public, having a contraceptive available that does not affect these aspects or that affects only in a low percentage of cases, would certainly increase the tolerability of the treatment.

The antiandrogenic profile of an OC can affect libido, mainly if the strong estrogenic activity increases SHBG levels, who plays a key role in the availability of androgens. The poor action of E2 on liver proteins, including SHBG, and the effect of E2 at a central and peripheral level, justify the optimal results with improvement of libido and sexuality obtained both during treatment with E2V/DNG [89] and when switching from a contraceptive with EE to a combination with E2/NOMAC [90].

Finally, the control and regularity of genital bleeding are two very important aspects in influencing the tolerability of the contraceptive. The fact that E2, compared to EE, has a very weak proliferative action at the endometrial level and, consequently, favors an unstable and easily bleeding endometrium, has for years limited the use of this estrogen in contraception. Today, however, the two OCs with E2 have been shown to have a substantially comparable profile to the OCs with EE as regards bleeding irregularities, with a progressive reduction in the appearance of spotting over time [74, 91]. Furthermore, contraception with E2, compared to that with EE, is associated with a reduction in the duration of withdrawal bleeding, with greater frequency with the absence of bleeding [74, 91], and these characteristics could also improve the woman's tolerability.

Author details

Anna Maria Paoletti[1*], Gian Benedetto Melis[1], Bruno Piras[2], Monica Pilloni[2], Pierina Zedda[3], Maria Francesca Marotto[2], Valerio Vallerino[4], Anna Melis[3], Valeria Taccori[3], Virginia Melis[3], Giulia Melis[3], Elena Giancane[5] and Manuela Neri[4]

1 Women's Wellness Foundation, Cagliari, Italy

2 University Hospital of Cagliari (UHC), Cagliari, Italy

3 University of Cagliari, Cagliari, Italy

4 Company of National Importance and High Specialization (CNIHS) G. Brotzu, Cagliari, Italy

5 San Martino Civil Hospital, Oristano, Italy

*Address all correspondence to: gineca.annapaoletti@tiscali.it

References

[1] Hassoun D. Natural family planning methods and barrier: CNGOF contraception guidelines. Gynecol Obstet Fertil Senol. 2018;**46**:873-882

[2] Trussel J. Contraceptive failure in the United States. Contraception. 2011;**83**:397-404

[3] Walsh TL, Frezieres RG, Peacock K, et al. Evaluation of the efficacy of a non-latex condom: Results from a randomized, controlled clinical trial. Perspectives on Sexual and Reproductive Health. 2003;**35**:79-86

[4] Boskey E. Polyisoprene Condoms for people with latex allergies. Verywell health.Available from: Verywellhealth.com/polypropene-condoms-for-people-with-latex-allergies-3132698. Updated on September 16, 2021

[5] Steiner MJ, Dominik R, Roundtree RW, et al. Contraceptive Effectiveness of a Polyurethane Condom and a Latex Condom: A Randomized Controlled Trial. Obstetrics and Gynecology. 2003;**101**:539-547

[6] Center for Disease Control (CDC). Condoms for prevention of sexually transmitted diseases. Morbidity and Mortality Weekly Report. 1988;**37**:133-137

[7] McNamee K. The female condom. Australian Family Physician. 2000;**29**:555-557

[8] Gilliam ML, Derman RJ. Barrier methods of contraception. Obstetrics and Gynecology Clinics of North America. 2000;**27**:841-858

[9] Secor R. The cervical cap. NAACOG's Clin. Issues. 1992;**3**:236-245

[10] Kreiss J, Ngugi E, Holmes K, et al. Efficacy of nonoxynol-9 contraceptive sponge use in preventing eterosexual acquisition of HIV in Nairobi prostitutes. JAMA. 1992;**268**:477-482

[11] Richardson B. Nonoxynol-9 as a vaginal microbicide for prevention of sexually transmitted infections: it's time to move on. Journal of the American Medical Association. 2002;**287**:1171-1172

[12] Ortiz ME, Croxatto HB, Bardin CW. Mechanisms of action of intrauterine devices. Obstetrical & Gynecological Survey. 1996;**51**:S42-S51

[13] Apter D, Gemzell-Danielsson K, et al. Pharmacokinetics of two low-dose levonorgestrel-releasing intrauterine systems and effects on ovulation rate and cervical function: Pooled analyses of phase II and III studies. Fertility and Sterility. 2014;**101**:1656-1662

[14] Gemzell-Danielsson K, Schellschmidt I, Apter D. A randomized, phase II study describing the efficacy, bleeding profile, and safety of two lowdose levonorgestrel-releasing intrauterine contraceptive systems and Mirena. Fertility and Sterility. 2012;**97**:616-622

[15] Fan G, Kang S, Ren M, et al. A single-arm phase III study exploring the efficacy and safety of LNG-IUS 8, a low-dose levonorgestrel intrauterine contraceptive system (total content 13.5 mg), in an Asia-Pacific population. Contraception. 2017;**95**:371-377

[16] Suvisaari J, Lähteenmäki P. Detailed analysis of menstrual bleeding patterns after postmenstrual and postabortal insertion of a copper IUD or a levonorgestrel-releasing intrauterine system. Contraception. 1996;**54**:201-208

[17] Rose S, Chaudhari A, Peterson CM. Mirena (Levonorgestrel Intrauterine system) a successful novel drug delivery option in contraception. Advanced Drug Delivery Reviews. 2009;**61**:808-812

[18] Nelson AL, Apter D, Hauck B, et al. Two low-dose levonorgestrel intrauterine contraceptive systems: A randomized controlled trial. Obstetrics and Gynecology. 2013;**122**:1205-1213

[19] Gemzell-Danielsson K, Buhling KJ, Dermout SM, et al. A phase III, single-arm study of LNG-IUS 8, a low-dose levonorgestrel intrauterine contraceptive system (total content 13.5 mg) in postmenarcheal adolescents. Contraception. 2016;**93**:507-512

[20] Cristobal I, Neyro J-L, Lete I. The new LNG-releasing IUS: A new opportunity to reduce the burden of unintended pregnancy. European Journal of Obstetrics, Gynecology, and Reproductive Biology. 2015;**190**:58-64

[21] Grandi G, Farulla A, Sileo FG, Facchinetti F. Levonorgestrel-releasing-intra-uterine systems as female contraceptives. Expert Opinion on Pharmacotherapy. 2018;**19**:677-686

[22] Curtis KM, Tepper NK, Jatlaoui TC, et al. U.S. medical eligibility criteria for contraceptive use, 2016. MMWR - Recommendations and Reports. 2016;**65**:1-103

[23] Goldin C, Katz LF. The power of the pill: Oral contraceptives and women's career and marriage decisions. Journal of Political Economy. 2002;**110**:730-770

[24] Canning D, Schultz TP. The economic consequences of reproductive health and family planning. The Lancet. 2012;**380**:165-171

[25] Cleland J, Conde-Agudelo A, Peterson H, et al. Contraception and health. The Lancet. 2012;**380**:149-156

[26] Black AY, Fleming NA, Rome ES. Pregnancy in adolescents. Adolescent medicine: state of the art reviews. 2012;**23**:123-138

[27] Jalanko E, Leppälahti S, Heikinheimo O, Gissler M. The risk of psychiatric morbidity following teenage induced abortion and childbirth-a longitudinal study from Finland. The Journal of Adolescent Health. 2020;**66**:345-351

[28] Cuomo A. Birth Control. Encyclopedia of Motherhood. Andrea O'Reilly. Thousand Oaks, California: Sage Publications; 2010

[29] Arisi E. La pillola che ha cambiato il mondo. Notiziario Gyneco AOGOI, numero. 2010;**5**:18-19

[30] Rott H. Contraception, venous thrombosis and biological plausibility. Minerva Medica. 2013;**104**:161-167

[31] deBastos M, Stegeman BH, Rosendaal FR, et al. Combined oral contraceptives: Venous thrombosis. Cochrane Database of Systematic Reviews. 2014;**3**:CD010813

[32] Lidegaard O, Lokkegaard E, Svendsen AL, Agger C. Hormonal contraception and risk of venous thromboembolism: National follow-up study. BMJ. 2009;**339**:b2890-b2899

[33] Lete I, Chabbert-Buffet N, Jamin C, et al. Haemostatic and metabolic impact of estradiol pills and drospirenone-containing ethinylestradiol pills vs. levonorgestrel-containing ethinylestradiol pills: A literature review. The European Journal of Contraception & Reproductive Health Care. 2015;**20**:329-343

[34] Sitruk-Ware R, Nath A. Characteristics and metabolic effects of estrogen and progestins contained

in oral contraceptive pills. Best Practice Res Clinic Endocrinol Metab. 2013;**27**:13-24

[35] James AH, Jamison MG, Brancazio LR, Myers ER. Venous thromboembolism during pregnancy and the postpartum period: Incidence, risk factors, and mortality. American Journal of Obstetrics and Gynecology. 2006;**194**:1311-1315

[36] Sitruk-Ware R, Nath A, Mishell DR Jr. Contraception technology: Past, present and future. Contraception. 2013;**87**:319-330

[37] Fruzzetti F, Bitzer J. Review of clinical experience with estradiol in combined oral contraceptives. Contraception. 2010;**81**:8-15

[38] Grandi G, Napolitano A, Cagnacci A. Metabolic impact of combined hormonal contraceptives containing estradiol. Expert Opinion on Drug Metabolism & Toxicology. 2016;**12**:779-787

[39] Neri M, Malune ME, Corda V, et al. Body composition and psychological improvement in healthy premenopausal women assuming the oral contraceptive containing micronized estradiol (E2) and nomegestrol acetate (NOMAC). Gynecological Endocrinology. 2017;**33**:958-962

[40] Grandi G, Xholli A, Napolitano A, et al. Prospective measurement of blood pressure and heart rate over 24 h in women using combined oral contraceptives with estradiol. Contraception. 2014;**90**:529-534

[41] Junge W, Mellinger U, Parke S, et al. Metabolic and haemostatic effects of estradiol valerate/dienogest, a novel oral contraceptive: A randomized, open-label, single-Centre study. Clinical Drug Investigation. 2011;**31**:573-584

[42] Ågren UM, Anttila M, Mäenpää-Liukko K, et al. Effects of a monophasic combined oral contraceptive containing nomegestrol acetate and 17β-oestradiol compared with one containing levonorgestrel and ethinylestradiol on haemostasis, lipids and carbohydrate metabolism. The European Journal of Contraception & Reproductive Health Care. 2011;**16**:444-457

[43] Dinger J, Do Minh T, Heinemann K. Impact of estrogen type on cardiovascular safety of combined oral contraceptives. Contraception. 2016;**94**:328-339

[44] Dinger J, Möhner S, Heinemann K. Combined oral contraceptives containing dienogest and estradiol valerate may carry a lower risk of venous and arterial thromboembolism compared to conventional preparations: Results from the extended INAS-SCORE study. Frontiers in Women's Health. 2020;**5**:1-8

[45] RCP Klaira®, Bayer S.p.A. - Milano https://farmaci.agenziafarmaco.gov.it/

[46] Christin-Maitre S, Serfaty D, Chabbert-Buffet N, et al. Comparison of a 24-day and a 21-day pill regimen for the novel combined oral contraceptive, nomegestrol acetate and 17β-estradiol (NOMAC/E2): A doubleblind, randomized study. Human Reproduction. 2011;**26**:1338-1347

[47] Kuhl H. Pharmacology of estrogens and progestogens: Influence of different routes of administration. Climacteric. 2005;**8**:3-63

[48] Ruan X, Seeger H, Mueck AO. The pharmacology of dienogest. Maturitas. 2012;**71**:337-344

[49] Guida M, Bifulco G, Di Spiezio SA, et al. Review of the safety, efficacy

and patient acceptability of the combined dienogest/estradiol valerate contraceptive pill. International Journal of Women's Health. 2010;**2**:279-290

[50] Klipping C, Duijkers I, Parke S, et al. Hemostatic effects of a novel estradiol-based oral contraceptive: An open-label, randomized, crossover study of estradiol valerate/dienogest versus ethinylestradiol/levonorgestrel. Drugs R D. 2011;**11**:159-170

[51] Lello S. Nomegestrol acetate: Pharmacology, safety profile and therapeutic efficacy. Drugs. 2010;**70**:541-559

[52] Gaussem P, Alhenc-Gelas M, Thomas JL, et al. Haemostatic effects of a new combined oral contraceptive, nomegestrol acetate/17β-estradiol, compared with those of levonorgestrel/ethinyl estradiol. A double-blind, randomised study. Thrombosis and Haemostasis. 2011;**105**:560-567

[53] Sørdal T, Grob P, Verhoeven C. Effects on bone mineral density of a monophasic combined oral contraceptive containing nomegestrol acetate/17β-estradiol in comparison to levonorgestrel/ethinylestradiol. Acta Obstetricia et Gynecologica Scandinavica. 2012;**91**:1279-1285

[54] Coelingh Bennink HJ, Holinka CF, Diczfalusy E. Estetrol review: Profile and potential clinical applications. Climacteric. 2008;**11**:47-58

[55] Holinka CF, Diczfalusy E, Coelingh Bennink HJ. Estetrol: a unique steroid in human pregnancy. The Journal of Steroid Biochemistry and Molecular Biology. 2008;**110**:138-143

[56] Kluft C, Zimmerman Y, Mawet M, et al. Reduced hemostatic effects with drospirenone-based oral contraceptives containing estetrol vs. ethinyl estradiol. Contraception. 2016;**pii:S0010-7824**:30398-30395

[57] Duijkers IJ, Klipping C, Zimmerman Y, et al. Inhibition of ovulation by administration of estetrol in combination with drospirenone or levonorgestrel: Results of a phase II dose-finding pilot study. The European Journal of Contraception & Reproductive Health Care. 2015;**20**:476-489

[58] Mawet M, Maillard C, Klipping C, et al. Unique effects on hepatic function, lipid metabolism, bone and growth endocrine parameters of estetrol in combined oral contraceptives. The European Journal of Contraception & Reproductive Health Care. 2015;**20**:463-475

[59] Creinin MD, Westhoff CL, Bouchard C, et al. Estetrol-drospirenone combination oral contraceptive: North American phase 3 efficacy and safety results. Contraception. 2021;**104**:222-228

[60] Cagnacci A, Ferrari S, Tirelli A, et al. Route of administration of contraceptives containing desogestrel/etonorgestrel and insulin sensitivity: A prospective randomized study. Contraception. 2009;**80**:34-39

[61] Galzote RM, Rafie S, Teal R, Mody SK. Transdermal delivery of combined hormonal contraception: A review of the current literature. International Journal of Women's Health. 2017;**9**:315-321

[62] Mansour D, Korver T, Marintcheva-Petrova M, Fraser IS. The effects of Implanon on menstrual bleeding patterns. The European Journal of Contraception & Reproductive Health Care. 2008;**13**(Suppl 1):13-28

[63] Archer DF, Ahrendt HJ, Drouin D. Drospirenone-only oral contraceptive:

Results from a multicenter noncomparative trial of efficacy, safety and tolerability. Contraception. 2015;**92**:439-444

[64] Duijkers IJM, Heger-Mahn D, Drouin D, Colli E, Skouby S. Maintenance of ovulation inhibition with a new progestogen-only pill containing drospirenone after scheduled 24-h delays in pill intake. Contraception. 2016;**93**:303-309

[65] Duijkers IJ, Heger-Mahn D, Drouin D. Skouby S a randomised study comparing the effect on ovarian activity of a progestogen-only pill (POP) containing desogestrel and a new POP containing drospirenone in a 24/4 regimen. The European Journal of Contraception & Reproductive Health Care. 2015;**20**:419-427

[66] Burkman R, Schlesselman JJ, Zieman M. Safety concerns and health benefits associated with oral contraception. American Journal of Obstetrics and Gynecology. 2004;**190**:S5-S22

[67] Iversen L, Sivasubramaniam S, Lee AJ, et al. Lifetime cancer risk and combined oral contraceptives: The Royal College of general Practitioners' Oral contraception study. American Journal of Obstetrics and Gynecology. 2017;**216**:580.e1-580.e9

[68] Iacovides S, Avidon I, Baker FC. What we know about primary dysmenorrhea today: A critical review. Human Reproduction Update. 2015;**21**:762-778

[69] Wong CL, Farquhar C, Roberts H, Proctor M. Oral contraceptive pill for primary dysmenorrhoea. Cochrane Database of Systematic Reviews. 2009;**4**:CD002120

[70] Strowitzki T, Kirsch B, Elliesen J. Efficacy of ethinylestradiol 20 μg/drospirenone 3 mg in a flexible extended regimen in women with moderate-to-severe primary dysmenorrhoea: An open-label, multicentre, randomised, controlled study. The Journal of Family Planning and Reproductive Health Care. 2012;**38**:94-101

[71] Grandi G, Napolitano A, Xholli A, et al. Effect of oral contraceptives containing estradiol and nomegestrol acetate or ethinyl-estradiol and chlormadinone acetate on primary dysmenorrhea. Gynecological Endocrinology. 2015;**31**:774-778

[72] Shimizu Y, Mita S, Takeuchi T, et al. Dienogest, a synthetic progestin, inhibits prostaglandin E2 production and aromatase expression by human endometrial epithelial cells in a spheroid culture system. Steroids. 2011;**76**:60-67

[73] Ray S, Ray A. Non-surgical interventions for treating heavy menstrual bleeding (menorrhagia) in women with bleeding disorders. Cochrane Database of Systematic Reviews. 2016;**11**:CD010338

[74] Ahrendt HJ, Makalová D, Parke S, et al. Bleeding pattern and cycle control with an estradiol-based oral contraceptive: A seven-cycle, randomized comparative trial of estradiol valerate/dienogest and ethinyl estradiol/levonorgestrel. Contraception. 2009;**80**:436-444

[75] Fraser IS, Römer T, Parke S, et al. Effective treatment of heavy and/or prolonged menstrual bleeding with an oral contraceptive containing estradiol valerate and dienogest: A randomized, double-blind phase III trial. Human Reproduction. 2011;**26**:2698-2708

[76] Fruzzetti F, Trémollieres F, Bitzer J. An overview of the development

of combined oral contraceptives containing estradiol: Focus on estradiol valerate/dienogest. Gynecological Endocrinology. 2012;**28**:400-408

[77] Ryu A, Kim TH. Premenstrual syndrome: A mini review. Maturitas. 2015;**82**:436-440

[78] Rapkin AJ, Akopians AL. Pathophysiology of premenstrual syndrome and premenstrual dysphoric disorder. Menopause International. 2012;**18**:52-59

[79] Sadler C, Smith H, Hammond J, et al. Southampton Women's survey study group. Lifestyle factors, hormonal contraception, and premenstrual symptoms: The United Kingdom Southampton Women's survey. Journal of Women's Health (2002). 2010;**19**:391-396

[80] Coffee AL, Kuehl TJ, Willis S, Sulak PJ. Oral contraceptives and premenstrual symptoms: Comparison of a 21/7 and extended regimen. American Journal of Obstetrics and Gynecology. 2006;**195**:1311-1319

[81] Sangthawan M, Taneepanichskul S. A comparative study of monophasic oral contraceptives containing either drospirenone 3 mg or levonorgestrel 150 microg on premenstrual symptoms. Contraception. 2005;**71**:1-7

[82] Witjes H, Creinin MD, Sundström-Poromaa I, et al. Comparative analysis of the effects of nomegestrol acetate/17 β-estradiol and drospirenone/ethinylestradiol on premenstrual and menstrual symptoms and dysmenorrhea. The European Journal of Contraception & Reproductive Health Care. 2015;**20**:296-307

[83] Saletu B. Sleep, vigilance and cognition in postmenopausal women: Placebo-controlled studies with 2 mg estradiol valerate, with and without 3 mg dienogest. Climacteric. 2003;**6**:37-45

[84] Hooper DJ. Attitudes, awareness, compliance and preferences among hormonal contraception users: A global, cross-sectional, self-administered, online survey. Clinical Drug Investigation. 2010;**30**:749-763

[85] Fruzzetti F, Perini D, Fornaciari L, et al. Discontinuation of modern hormonal contraceptives: An Italian survey. The European Journal of Contraception & Reproductive Health Care. 2016;**21**:449-454

[86] Peipert JF, Zhao Q, Allsworth JE, et al. Continuation and satisfaction of reversible contraception. Obstetrics and Gynecology. 2011;**117**:1105-1113

[87] Rosenstock JR, Peipert JF, Madden T, et al. Continuation of reversible contraception in teenagers and young women. Obstetrics and Gynecology. 2012;**120**:1298-1305

[88] American Academy of Pediatrics. Policy statement. Contraception for adolescents: Committee on adolescence. Pediatrics. 2014;**134**:e1244-e1256

[89] Caruso S, Agnello C, Romano M, et al. Preliminary study on the effect of four-phasic estradiol valerate and dienogest (E2V/DNG) oral contraceptive on the quality of sexual life. The Journal of Sexual Medicine. 2011;**8**:2841-2850

[90] Caruso S, Cianci S, Cariola M, et al. Improvement of low sexual desire due to Antiandrogenic combined Oral contraceptives after switching to an Oral contraceptive containing 17β-Estradiol. Journal of Women's Health (2002). 2017;**26**:728-734

[91] Mansour D, Verhoeven C, Sommer W, et al. Efficacy and

DOI: http://dx.doi.org/10.5772/intechopen.111643

tolerability of a monophasic combined oral contraceptive containing nomegestrol acetate and 17β-oestradiol in a 24/4 regimen, in comparison to an oral contraceptive containing ethinylestradiol and drospirenone in a 21/7 regimen. The European Journal of Contraception & Reproductive Health Care. 2011;**16**:430-443

Chapter 4

Contraception and Family Planning: New Aspects Related to the Therapeutic Possibilities

Vincenzina Bruni and Metella Dei

Abstract

The therapeutic use of CHC (combined hormonal contraception) is examined in healthy patients who accept this contraceptive method and in patients with specific problems (abundant menstrual flows, hyperandrogenism, chronic pelvic pain, PMS, disability, different lifestyles, etc.) who require contraception. Rational motivation for the non-only contraceptive use of this device is represented by their mechanism of action: antigonadotropic action with ovulatory block and reduced production of sex steroids, endometrial response with changes in menstrual bleeding, action on the progesterone receptor, downregulation of estrogen receptors, and anti-inflammatory action. The dosing regimen (continuous regimen) can also modulate the therapeutic response in relation to the utilization in pathologies with catamenial exacerbation. The metabolic response varies in relation to the characteristics of the association (synthetic or natural estrogen, progestin component) with possible hepatocellular action, characteristic for associations with EE. Numerous data on associations with EE, few data with natural estrogens are available; the assumptions of use in relation to particular therapeutic lines are examined.

Keywords: combined hormonal contraceptives, endometrium, bleedings, endometriosis, hyperandrogenism

1. Introduction

Today, the panorama of combined hormonal contraception includes association of ethinyl-estradiol or natural estrogens (estradiol valerate, estradiol, estetrol) with various progestogens. All the associations share the ability to inhibit ovulation by antigonadotropic action with reduction of follicular activity and, consequently, steroid production. This effect modifies endometrial response in variable ways depending on the characteristics of the estrogen and the type of progestogen used. The metabolic impact of CHC (combined hormonal contraception) is also different.

1.1 Associations with ethinyl estradiol (EE)

This synthetic estrogen (**Figure 1**) is delivered by oral, transdermal, and vaginal route, with rapid and complete absorption. Its half-life is 26 ± 7 hrs. Binding affinity with Sex Hormone Binding Globulin is low; binding to albumin is 98.5% effective; bioavailability is 45–55%. The molecule's high metabolic stability is due to the presence of the C = CH group, which prevents the oxidation of 17β and the transformation into estrone. The oxidation of the C=CH group by cytochrome P 450 3 A 4 induces the formation of an intermediate metabolite capable of inhibiting the same cytochrome P 450 3 A 4. This results in accumulation that explains the greater biological potency of EE compared to E2 in all estrogen-related activities, in particular the synthesis of certain hepatic proteins, such as SHBG, the increase of which is dependent on the dose of EE and the type of progestin used. Metabolization at the gastric level is modest (0.44%); more than 30% of EE is sulfated in the intestine (during fasting), while endogenous estrogens are glucuronide conjugates [1].

It is known that progestogens stimulate endometrial 17-beta HSD2, which inactivates estradiol in the endometrial cell, reducing local estrogenic effect. This does not happen for EE, which inhibits the action of this enzyme [2]. This leads to relative endometrial stability for associations with EE. Concerning metabolic impact, EE is characterized by its dose-dependent hepatocellular action, which is modulated by the associated progestin (**Figure 2**). The progestogen component differs in half-life, progestogen potency, residual androgenic activity or antiandrogenic character, neuroprotective and anti-mineralocorticoid action, and glucocorticoid action with different metabolic repercussions [3].

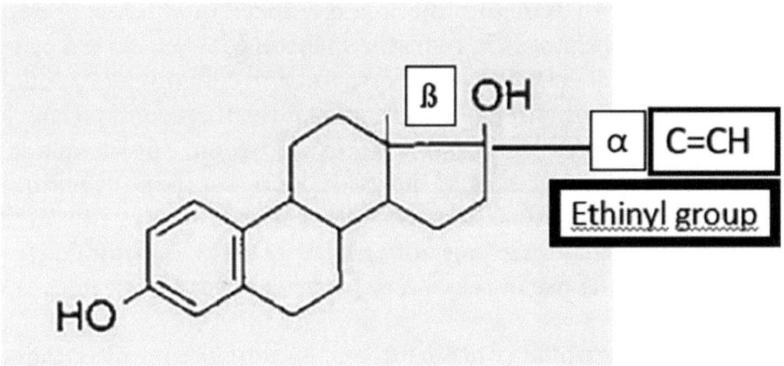

Figure 1.
Ethinyl-estradiol.

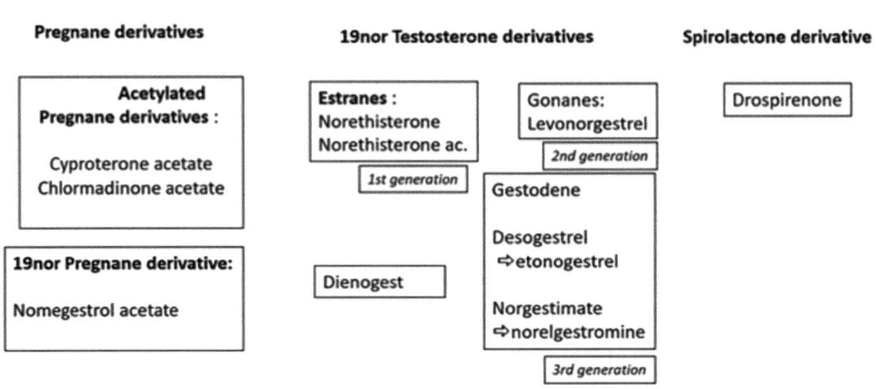

Figure 2.
Progestogens in contraceptive combinations with Ethynylestradiol.

Progestogens with residual androgenic activity moderate the prothrombotic activity of EE. Combinations with levonorgestrel (LNG) and norgestimate (NGS) are at lower VTE risk [4]. In particular, LNG has an androgenic activity of 3–4% and an anabolic activity of 20–30% that of testosterone. Its half-life (in association with EE) is 36 +/− 13 hours. The binding of LNG to SHBG is 50%. LNG does not induce a significant increase of SHBG when associated with EE. Norgestimate is a prodrug with rapid metabolism into Norelgestromin (NGMN), 39% in the liver and 49% in the intestinal mucosa. During hepatic first pass, 25% is metabolized to LNG, and at a later time, liver microsome activity produces a further 10% of LNG [5]. In a study [6] on 12 volunteers, about 22.6% of the dose of NGM administered in association with EE became systemically available as LNG. The progestogenic activity of norgestimate is marked, the androgenic activity minimal. There is glucocorticoid antagonist activity, albeit modest, and moderate mineralocorticoid antagonist activity. The binding of NGM to albumin is 99%, no binding to SHBG. From the point of view of therapeutic use, antiandrogenic activity of progestins, that is, the antagonism on androgen receptor (synergic with the inhibitory action of skin 5a reductase), is a relevant feature of biological action. This action is typical of cyproterone acetate, dienogest (40% compared to CPA), drospirenone (30% compared tp CPA), chlormadinone acetate, and, minimally, nomegestrol acetate (NOMAC) [7].

All the progestins used in contraception have a central action. They probably have an effect on the hypothalamic Kisspeptin-Neurokinin-Dynorphin neuronal system that regulates GnRH secretion and gonadotropin production. We do not know if the inhibitory action is direct or mediated by endogenous opiates. This effect requires estrogen priming and entails ovulation inhibition [8]. At the peripheral level, all progestins present in combined oral contraception (COC) induce decidualization of endometrium, albeit to different degrees. This effect is documented *in vitro* by morphological changes and is mediated by the interaction with progesterone receptors and enhanced, during COC use, by the progestin from the first days of intake of the combination drug. Progestins (LNG, NETA, DNG, DRSP, MPA) have been demonstrated to exercise anti-inflammatory activity, above all in the endometrium and peritoneum. Various studies have evidenced its ability to inhibit the production of prostaglandins, as well as to modulate pro- and anti-inflammatory cytokines, and regulate T-cell activation, resulting in reduced tissue production of nerve growth factors and vascular growth factors. The inhibition of proliferative signaling pathways mediated by estrogen receptor beta also plays a role [9]. These effects have been extensively documented in women with endometriosis as well as in healthy controls [10].

1.2 Associations with natural estrogens

Combinations of estradiol valerate with dienogest, estradiol with NOMAC, and estetrol with drospirenone are available.

17β Estradiol valerate (E2V) is the esterified form of 17ß-Estradiol (E2). E2V is rapidly and completely absorbed and hydrolyzed to natural estradiol during the first passage in the gastrointestinal tract. E2V is almost identical to E2 in terms of pharmacokinetics, and exactly identical in pharmacodynamics and clinic. The assessment of estradiol levels during E2V therapy puts in evidence that 1 mg of E2V is equivalent to 0.76 mg of E2 [11]. Regarding pharmacokinetics, 38% of estradiol is bound to SHBG, 60% to albumin, and 2–3% circulates in free form. The production of SHBG is increased by 150% after 28 days of intake. About 95% of estradiol undergoes metabolization before entering the systemic circulation. Its main metabolites are estrone, estrone sulfate, and estrone glucuronide. Estradiol has a terminal half-life of 13–20 hours due to enterohepatic recirculation and the pool of circulating estrogen sulfates and glucuronides; its plasma half-life of estradiol is 90 minutes [12].

Estetrol (E4), a natural estrogen with four hydroxyl group, is synthetized by the human fetal liver only during pregnancy (**Figure 3**). Detectable blood levels are present at 9 weeks of gestation with exponential increase during pregnancy. The fetal exposure at term of pregnancy is about 3 mg/day, comparable with oral treatment with 50–60 mgE4 per day.

E4 half-life is 28–30 hours. The stimulus on liver SHBG synthesis is reduced. It also inhibits ovulation at a dosage of 5, 10, 20 mg due to a combination of central and peripheral action (given its suppressive effect on the ERα membrane). This effect is more pronounced using 20 mg doses [13]. E4 is able to block membrane ER and at the same time to activate nuclear ER exerting a strong estrogenic effect. E4 is an estrogenic agonist in the vagina [14], myometrium, endometrium, central nervous system, and bone. A dose-dependent proliferative effect has been shown in the endometrium in animal models [15] with increased cell differentiation, rather than mitotic activity [16]; dose-dependent increases in uterine weight were also seen. In combination with E2, estetrol has an anti-estrogenic action on breast tissue [17], and it exercises neuroprotective and antioxidant action in the CNS [18, 19] (**Table 1**).

Dienogest is a 19-nortestosterone derivative, that is, with 17a-ethinyl group (as in levonorgestrel) replaced by a 17a-cyanomethyl group. Despite limited *in vitro* binding affinity (approximately 10%) to the progesterone receptor in human uterine tissue, it is characterized *in vivo* by a potent endometrial activity, after oral intake. It follows that circulating dienogest levels are relatively high compared with those found with

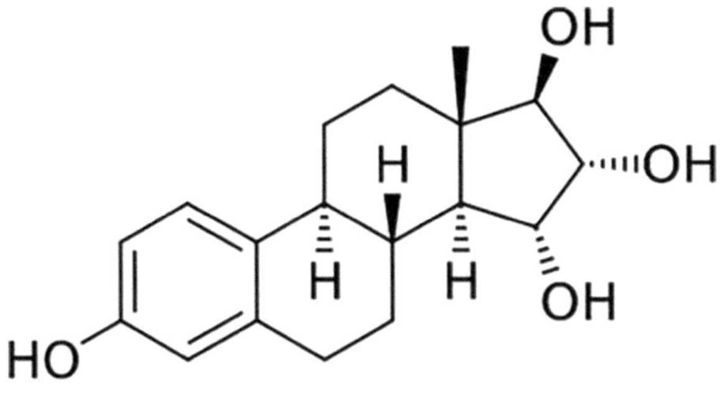

Figure 3.
Estetrol.

	E2V /DNG	E2/NOMAC	E4/DRSP
Half-life progestin (hours)	11	> 45	30
Antigonadotrope activity	moderate	strong	good
Progestational activity	strong	strong	good
Antiandrogenic activity	40% compared to CPA	15% compared to CPA	30% compared to CPA
Antimineralocorticoid activity	/	/	significant

Table 1.
Main characteristics of progestins in association with natural estrogens [20–22]. Half-life and biological activities of progestins used in COC with natural estrogens.

similar oral doses of others progestins [23, 24]. The endometrial action is carried out by blocking the aromatase, and by inhibiting COX_2 and the synthesis of PGE2, with consequent reduced production of estrogens, increased cellular apoptosis, and impaired angiogenesis [25–27].

Nomegestrol acetate NOMAC is a 9 norprogesterone derivate; it is devoid of estrogenic, androgenic, glucocorticoid, and mineralocorticoid activity but displays an anti-estrogenic activity on the endometrium and a moderate antiandrogenic activity [28]. It has a strong endometrial activity and a high contraceptive efficacy due to its high antigonadotropic effect and long elimination half-life [29].

Drospirenone (DRSP) is a spirolactone derivative with anti-mineralocorticoid activity. We remind that in addition to the kidney, there are several other cells and organs expressing mineral corticoid receptors, as blood vessels, inflammatory and immune cells, adipose tissue, and central nervous system [30]. So DRSP reduces differentiation of adipocytes, facilitates endothelial response to damage, and modulates inflammatory reactions. It also exerts neuroactive properties, balancing the negative effects of glucocorticoids on neurons and glia cells, and increasing the production of endogenous opiates [31, 32]. DRSP does not exert glucocorticoid activity as well as estrogenic activity. In ectopic endometrium, it shows anti-inflammatory effects [33].

The bleeding profile of the three associations with natural estrogens is presented in **Table 2** [34–39]. All of them induce a reduction of menstrual blood loss. Note that the association E4—DRSP seems favorable in terms of expected menstrual cycle and intermenstrual bleedings.

Concerning endometrial histology during the use of these combinations, a study on E2V/DNG put in evidence, after 20 cycles of use, only 11.4% of proliferative, and 16.9% of secretory endometrium vs. 64% of atrophic or inactive endometrium [40]. No specific data are available for E2/NOMAC association, even if clinical data support a strong endometrial activity. E4/DRSP induces, after 7 cycles, 81% of atrophic or inactive endometrium, 5% of secretory, and 22% of proliferative endometrium [41].

The pharmacological properties and the biological activities of these steroid combinations explain the possibilities of a therapeutic use.

	E2V /DNG	E2/NOMAC [34]	E4/DRSP [35]
Expected menstrual cycle	European Study: 77.7–83.2% [36]	82% 2nd cycle	76.5% 1st cycle
	North American Study: 76.5% [37]	68% 12th cycle	87% 12th cycle
			91–9 – 94.4%
Menstrual bleeding duration (days)	European Study:4.7–4	1.9–2.5	≤ 2 gg
	North American Study: 4.1–4-7	3.1–3.3	
Intermenstrual bleedings	European Study:28.8% (1st cycle)-11.25% (11th CYCLE)	> 20% reduction over time	13–17.4% (1st cycle)
	North American Study: 14%		16.2–19-8% (13th cycle)

Table 2.
Bleeding patterns during use of natural estrogen combinations.

2. Heavy menstrual bleeding (HMB)

We define excessive menstrual bleeding as blood loss of more than 80 ml (pad change every 1–2 hours, the presence of significant clots, and a duration of more than 8 days). Sometimes they represent a real clinical emergency. The rationale of using CHC is the association among the anti-ovulatory effect, with inhibition of follicular activity and ovarian steroid production, the suppression of endometrial proliferation, and the precocious decidualization, with reduction of menstrual flow.

In acute HMB, the treatment must start after excluding pregnancy complications. When it is possible, an anamnestic and US evaluation to rule out organic pathology is useful. As we have explained in the previous paragraph, a more rapid cessation of bleeding and greater endometrial stability are ensured using combinations with EE. In hemorrhagic menarche with 8–10 g/dL of hemoglobin levels, the use of monophasic COCs containing 30–50 mcg EE, given once every 6 hours for 2–4 days, followed by the same dose given every eight hours for three days and then every 12 hours for the next 14 days, is recommended [42]. The extensive experience has been confirmed by a recent revision [43]. In clinical practice, the dosage of EE should be individualized in relation to symptoms, entity of bleeding, and patient BMI. The same therapeutic option is possible even in the presence of a hemorragic diathesis. The guidelines for the treatment in patients with von Willebrandt disease from the National Heart, Lung, and Blood Institute stated that the first choice of therapy for HMB should be COC, with LNG-IUs as the second choice [43].

In cases of contraindications to COC, MPA (150 mg im) followed by oral MPA therapy (20 mg 3 times daily X 1 week) or oral NETA (40 mg daily, in multi dose/week) are proposed. The response is slightly lower with progestins than with COC use. A recent study [44] has pointed out as the estrogen-containing treatment for HMB (20, 30, or 35 mcg of EE as monotherapy or in a COC) initiated within 3 months of menarche was associated with reduced growth at 24 months compared to progesterone-only or nonhormonal methods. Authors invited to a particular attention in case of subjects with short stature at baseline.

Regarding chronic HBM, there is strong evidence supporting the impact of COCs on reducing menstrual bleeding volumes and unscheduled bleedings [45]. A recent Cochrane review [46] from 8 RCT involving 805 women has demonstrated the varied but positive response to COC, with improvement in 12–77% of subjects compared to only 3% of those on placebo. The data regarding E2V/DNG association demonstrate a reduction of blood loss from 65 to 80% after only a single treatment cycle in women with HMB and in women with normal menstrual cycles [47–49]. The association E2/NOMAC is also characterized by a significant reduction in menstrual blood loss [39, 50].

3. Endometriosis

Endometriosis is an estrogen-dependent chronic inflammatory disease, related to the presence of ectopic endometrial glandular epithelium and stroma. The endometriotic tissue shows few differences from the eutopic endometrium. First of all, epigenetic modifications of estrogen receptor have been demonstrated with the reduction of ERα (physiological inductor of progesterone receptor) and increase in ERβ. The induction of progesterone receptor is reduced, with prevalence of PRA, which is less active than PRB. As a consequence, the production of 17βOH steroid dehydrogenase type 2, which entails the conversion of E2 to E1, is reduced. Aromatase activity is enhanced, with increased production of estrogens from androgenic precursors. So, in endometriotic implants, hyper-estrogenism associated with resistance to progesterone is present [51]. The activation of inflammatory response and the dysfunction of immune response participate in the stimulation of angiogenesis, neurogenesis, and fibrogenesis, modulated by estrogens. As a consequence, the effects of COC on eutopic and ectopic endometrium, mainly the reduction of estrogen receptors induced by activation of PB receptors and increased metabolization of estradiol into estrone, are not the same in ectopic endometrium. In endometriotic implants, the predominant presence of βE receptors and the marked reduction of PB receptors counteract the decidualization.

The current Endometriosis Guidelines [52] recommend (as strong recommendation) hormone treatment with CHC (oral, vaginal ring, or transdermal) or progestogens to reduce endometriosis-associated pain. Various mechanisms explain the efficacy of CHC as a therapeutic intervention. The antigonadotropic effect reduces ovarian follicular activity and steroid production, containing menstrual bleeding, retrograde flux, and peritoneal inflammatory state. The absence of ovulation also plays a role, because we know that the follicular fluid of women with endometriosis contains elevated estrogen levels, which stimulate the proliferation of endometrial implants more than peritoneal fluid [53]. The CHCs demonstrate a dominant progestative effect on the endometrium, dependent on the length of use of the association. A downregulation of estrogen receptors with inhibition of cellular proliferation has been demonstrated, together with the stimulus of progesterone receptors [54]. The inhibition of endometrial metalloproteases and the anti-inflammatory action exerted by the progestogen component are complementary to the hormonal effects.

All the contraceptive associations with 20 or 30 mcg of EE associated with various progestins are effective for the relief of endometriosis-related dysmenorrhea, pelvic pain and dyspareunia, and improve quality of life, but the entity of the response is variable [55–57]. The vaginal ring that releases 15mcg of EE and 120 mg of etonogestrel (active metabolite of desogestrel) has also been used in the treatment of chronic pelvic pain of pre-surgical and post-surgical endometriosis. The rationale for use relates to the reduced steroid systemic concentrations compared with the oral route and the possible advantages of the drug prompt administration with direct effect on deep infiltrating endometriosis. One study involving 207 young women [58] compered 123 vaginal ring wearers and 84 patch wearers (EE 20 mcg and Norelgestromin 150 mcg). A reduction of symptoms was evident in both treatment groups, with greater efficacy in the use of the ring in patients with recto-vaginal lesions. A randomized, prospective study [59] on 60 women with chronic pelvic pain treated with vaginal ring in continuous regimen for 84 days or with COC with EE 30 mcg and LNG 150 mcg showed that the two treatments are equally effective. Compliance, satisfaction, and acceptance to use were higher in ring users (80%) than in COC users (70%).

According to a systematic review [60], a certain persistence of symptoms under estrogen-progestin treatment is present in 59% of cases, as well as the relapse of pelvic pain in 17% of cases at follow-up. The studies reported do not consent a specific correlation between type of endometriotic lesions and therapeutical results, although subjects with peritoneal endometriosis or ovarian endometrioma could probably be more easily treated than those with profound infiltrative lesions [61]. However, significant improvement in pain symptoms, menstrual bleeding, and sexual quality of life was also reported in patients with deep-infiltrating endometriosis (DIE) with or without associated adenomyosis after treatment with EE 30 mcg/DNG 2 mg [62].

There is some debate about whether or not a more competent choice of the COC could give better results. Considering the characteristics of the associations, an elevated progestative activity and a reduced estrogenic stimulation have been proposed [63], because we know that estrogens promote inflammatory reactions, neurogenesis, and angiogenesis inside the endometriotic lesions. This could orient the choice versus low EE dosages or the use of natural estrogen associations. We note that, even if the differences in pharmacokinetic do not consent calculation of clear equivalence, in relation to various metabolic and hemostatic parameter, it has been proposed that 2 mg of estradiol should be considered similar to 5 to 10 mcg of ethynyl-estradiol. The interindividual differences in drug efficacy and metabolism must also be considered. Choice of associations with these characteristics is based on speculative consideration and not on specific clinical trials, but there are favorable data on the use of natural estrogen combinations. The combination E2V/DNG has also been used in the treatment of endometriosis, resulting in a better reduction of pelvic pain and an improvement of the QoL compared to NSAIDS [64]. Experiences involving small groups have been published also using estradiol/NOMAC association with reduction of painful symptoms and size of ovarian endometriomas; DIE lesions remained stable [65] and showed better results than using NSAIDs [66].

There are no data available on the use of the E4/DRSP combination in treatment of endometriosis, but some experimental data deserve a mention. A recent *in vitro* study [67] on the effects of E4 on epithelial and stromal endometriotic cells evidenced no modification of cell viability or proliferation at any concentrations. Considering steroid receptor effect, both the ratio ERα/ERβ and PR increased (further by activation of PR-related genes) with possible beneficial effect. In comparison, during 17β estradiol use, there is an increase of cell number and reduction in apoptosis, without modification of ERα/ERβ ratio. The association with drospirenone could also be beneficial. One study [33] demonstrated the anti-inflammatory effect of DRSP with DNA synthesis decrease in stromal cells and significant reduction of IL-6, IL-8, VEGF, and NGF mRNA expression in endometriotic tissues obtained from patients that had undergone laparoscopic surgery for endometrioma.

Studies comparing COC with EE and various progestins with dienogest alone showed that compliance and side effects were similar, but the improvement of pain symptoms resulted superior with DNG in all the studies (**Table 3**) [68–73].

It has been widely demonstrated that the use of COCs decreases the risk of disease recurrence after conservative surgery. In a randomized pilot study related to postoperative administration of DNG or COC (EE 30 μg/LNG 0.3 mg) compared to placebo, self-reported pain was found reduced in both treatment groups after 6 months of treatment [74]. In another trial, postoperative administration of E2V/DNG for 9 months or GnRH for 6 months seemed equally effective in preventing pelvic pain recurrence in the first 9 months of follow-up [75]. There is insufficient evidence, however, to reach definitive conclusions about the superiority of any particular treatment: all hormonal regimens (cyclic or continuous COC, GnRHa, DNG, LNG-IUS, GnRHa + OC, and GnRHa + LNG-IUS) given as long-term treatment tend to reduce the risk of endometrioma recurrence [76]. Similar results were obtained in another systematic review and meta-analysis [77]: Hormonal suppression immediately after surgery was able to reduce recurrence of pain. The study was related to monophasic and multiphasic COC use in cyclic or continuous regimen, LNG IUS, and Dienogest 2 mg.

Combinations	Design of the study	End points	Results	Ref.
EE 30 mcg/DRSP 3 mg (flexible extended regimen) compared to DNG 2 mg	Randomized clinical trial	Pelvic pain, QoL	DNG more effective	[68]
EE 30 mcg/DRSP 3 mg (24 weeks) compared to DNG 2 mg	Randomized clinical trial	Pelvic pain, dysmenorrhea, dyspareunia, QoL	No significant differences DNG fewer side effect	[69]
EE 20 mcg/LNG 100 mg (continuous regimen) compared to DNG 2 mg	Prospective cohort study	Size of endometriomas	DNG more effective	[70]
		DIE, pain, QoL		
EE 30 mcg/DNG 2 mg compared to DNG 2 mg	Multicentric case-control study	Size of endometriomas; pain	DNG more effective	[71]
			No statistical difference in reduction pain symptoms	
EE 30 mcg/DNG 2 mg compared to DNG 2 mg	Observational study	Pain, QoL, and sexual satisfaction	DNG more effective reduction over time.	[72]
E2 1.5 mg /NOMAC 2.5 mg compared to DNG 2 mg	Randomized study	Pain, QoL, and sexual function	DNG more effective	[73]

Table 3.
Overview of the available comparative data of using COC compared to DNG 2 mg.

The treatment choice should be individualized according to each woman's needs. One important issue regards the comorbidities associated with endometriosis. An observational study pointed out that women with endometriosis had an elevated prevalence of psychiatric disorders and significant association with pain severity [78]. A meta-analysis of 24 studies (99,614 women) showed, in particular, higher levels of depression among women with endometriosis compared to controls [79]. The association was largely determined by chronic pain [80] but was also modulated by individual and context vulnerabilities. The impact of COC and progestins on the risk of depression should be considered. The data in the literature are controversial [81]. A significant association [82–85], no association [86–89], or improvement of mood have been reported [90, 91].

Moreover, migraine may be associated with dysmenorrhea and endometriosis [92]. The prevalence of migraine especially in advanced stages of endometriosis is significantly higher compared with controls [93], and this is confirmed also in adolescents [94]. Thus, the presence of aura should be investigated, and an appropriate choice of COC is necessary. Hemorrhagic diathesis is a risk factor for endometriotic implants and could require a specific choice of COC or an extended regimen in order to avoid acyclic bleeding.

4. Adenomyosis

Adenomyosis is defined by the presence of endometrial implants inside the myometrium. The rationale for using COCs in adenomyosis is related to the induced decidualization and subsequent atrophy of the endometrium, also in adenomyotic foci [95], reducing pain, abnormal bleedings, and uterine volume [96]. Abnormal uterine bleedings are not pathognomonic of adenomyosis, although an increased severity of the disease may increase the likelihood of this symptom [97]. COC is less effective in controlling pain and bleeding than LNG-IUS [98] or oral DNG [99].

5. Hyperandrogenism

Androgen excess can be characterized by specific clinical features associated or not with biochemical hyperandrogenism. A clinical evaluation is important to differentiate skin symptoms of androgen excess (hirsutism, acne, seborrhea, and female-pattern hair loss) from states of virilization (clitoris hypertrophy, voice modifications, increase in muscle mass, baldness, and mammary gland atrophy) related to more severe adrenal or ovarian diseases. Clinical hyperandrogenism is often associated with menstrual irregularities (chronic oligomenorrhea, amenorrhea, dysfunctional uterine bleeding) and metabolic dysfunction (as in polycystic ovary syndrome).

The motivation for therapeutic use of COC in hyperandrogenism is multifactorial: suppression of ovarian androgen production (and for few progestins also adrenal androgen production), SHBG increase, 5α reductase activity inhibition, and competition for skin androgen receptors with some combinations (**Table 4**).

The inhibition of ovarian steroid production is related to the anti-ovulatory effect, typical of all COCs. The circulating levels of SHBG, and consequently the amount of testosterone bound and inactive, are dependent on the type of estrogen and the progestogen present in the association. The liver production of SHBG is induced in a dose-dependent manner by EE, but it is also conditioned by the progestogen associated. COCs containing second generation progestins (with a minimal residual androgenicity) and/or the lower estrogen doses (20–25 μg EE) were found to have less impact on SHBG concentrations [100]. It is less evident with associations containing natural estrogens. For instance, SHBG plasma levels decreased with E4 (5, 10, or 20 mg) in association with LNG, while they showed a dose-dependent slight increase with 5 or 10 mg E4 in association with DRSP. This increase is considerably less than with the combination EE/DRSP [22, 101] (**Table 5**).

Concerning acne, it is a complex and multifactorial inflammatory disease involving excessive and altered sebum production, cutaneous dysbiosis, abnormalities of

Cyproterone acetate	Dienogest	Norgestimate	Drospirenone	Chlormadinone acetate	Nomegestrol acetate
Half-life 50 hrs	Half-life 11 hrs	Half-life 45–71 hrs	Half-life 30 hrs	Half-life 34–39 hrs	Half-life 50 hrs
CPA 2 mg/ EE 35 mcg 21 + 7	DNG 2 mg / EE 30 mcg 21 + 7; 24 + 4	NGM 250 mg/ EE 35 mcg 21 + 7	DRSP 3 mg/ EE 30 mcg 21 + 7	CMA 3 mg/ EE 30 mcg 21 + 7	NOMAC 2.5 mg/ E2 1.5 mg 24 + 4
	DNG 2–3 mg/ E2V 3–2-1 mg quadriphasic	NGM 180 mg-215 mg/ EE 35 mcg Triphasic	DRSP 3 mg/ EE 20 mcg 21 + 7; 24 + 4		

Table 4.
Progestins with antiandrogenic or non-androgenic activity in COC.

Androgen production suppression	SHBG increase	5a reductase activity inhibition	Androgen receptor competition
Specific types or doses of progestins, estrogens, or EP combinations	Higher increase in COCs with EE and non-androgenic progestins	Related to the type of progestins: *in vitro* evaluation compared to finasteride:	Anti-androgenic progestins
cannot currently be recommended → similar efficacy in treating hirsutism [102]	Moderate increase in COCs with natural estrogens	3-keto desogestrel cyproterone acetate ↓ dienogest levonorgestrel norgestimate [103]	(**Table 4**) Less metabolic impact

Table 5.
Rationale for the therapeutic effect of COCs on hyperandrogenism.

proliferation and differentiation of keratinocytes of the pilo-sebaceous unit, and activation of the inflammatory and the innate immune responses [104]. The influence of the hormonal milieu is relevant, but it is not the main cause, even if the androgenic effect on sebocytes differentiation and on lipogenesis has been well documented [105], and increased androgen production plays a recognized role in the pathogenesis of adult acne [104]. COCs are an important therapeutic aid in treating acne manifestations but in synergy with dermatological therapies.

A frequent and particular condition of hyperandrogenism is polycystic ovary syndrome (PCOS), an endocrinopathy characterized by irregular menstrual cycles, hyper-androgenism, characteristic ovarian morphology, systemic chronic inflammatory state, and dysmetabolism. A wide phenotypic variability is typical, ranging from mild hirsutism and anovulation to menstrual disorders, heavy signs of hyperandrogenism, and overweight. It is important to point out that the metabolic component worsens the androgen excess and should be investigated and treated, together with endocrine disorders.

In the report from the Multidisciplinary Androgen Excess and PCOS Committee [104], COCs in association with topical therapy are the first line of therapy in mild, moderate, or severe acne with hyperandrogenism. Estro-progestins may be used also in non-hyperandrogenic patients with moderate or severe adult acne as second-line therapy. Various combinations have been used: ethynyl-estradiol associated with acetylated pregnane-derivatives (CPA, CMA), 19 nor testosterone progestins (LNG, GSD, DSG/ETG, NGSM), and spironolactone derivative (DRSP). All COCs were effective on acne, but less androgenic progestins should be preferred. Moreover, a real therapeutic effect on hirsutism requires association with antiandrogens and, in some cases, esthetic procedures. Considering subjects with PCOS, COCs represent an effective and safe treatment in women with any PCOS phenotype. For patients with metabolic risk, overweight, or moderate insulin resistance that does not require insulin-sensitizer use, lifestyle changes should be promoted. The association with metformin has been widely used in subjects with relevant dysmetabolism [106]. A combination with natural estrogens [107] has demonstrated a positive influence on acne in a small number of patients (improvement in 52.8% and worsening 3.8% after 12 months of therapy).

Current guidelines [108] recommend the following:

- The COCs alone should be recommended in adult women with PCOS for management of hyperandrogenism and/or irregular menstrual cycles.
- The COCs alone should be considered in adolescents with a clear diagnosis of PCOS for the management of clinical hyperandrogenism and/or irregular menstrual cycles.
- The COCs could be considered in adolescents who are deemed "at risk" but not yet diagnosed with PCOS, for the management of clinical hyperandrogenism and irregular menstrual cycles.

COCs as monotherapy are not very effective in arresting mild to moderate alopecia or hirsutism and are preferably combined with an anti-androgen to achieve a better response when targeting hirsutism and hair loss [109]. A longitudinal study [110] has documented the progressive reduction of Ferriman-Gallway score obtained with the association EE-35/CPA 2 mg > in 18% of cases after 6 cycles of treatment, in 55% of cases after 24 cycles, and in 72% of cases after 48 cycles.

6. Conclusion

The therapeutic use of COCs in various clinical conditions (not all specifically examined in this chapter) should always consider individual risk factors and the eligibility criteria for contraceptive use. The pharmacological knowledge, which motivates benefits, is also the prerequisite for understanding the eventual risks.

The thrombotic risk is linked to the hepatocellular action of EE; it is dose-dependent and limited by the association with progestins with residual androgenic activity (LNG). The combinations with Norgestimate, non-androgenic progestins (but to be considered a prodrug for its metabolization in Norelgestromin and LGN) are recognized in various systematic review and meta-analyses at low thrombotic risk [111–115]. Current epidemiological data on COCs with natural estrogens show a comparable risk to the association of EE-LNG [116, 117].

The choice of combination, even for therapeutic use, cannot disregard a careful familial and personal evaluation of the subject and, if possible, the correction of metabolic risk factors present.

Author details

Vincenzina Bruni[1*] and Metella Dei[2]

1 University of Florence, Florence, Italy

2 Ob Gyn and Endocrinology, Florence, Italy

*Address all correspondence to: vbruni.prof@gmail.com

References

[1] Back DJ, Madden S, Orme EM. Gastrointestinal metabolism of contraceptive steroids. American Journal of Obstetrics and Gynecology. 1990;**163**: 2138-2145

[2] Gurpide E, Marks C. Influence of endometrial 17b-hydroxysteroid dehydrogenase activity on the binding of estradiol to receptors. The Journal of Clinical Endocrinology and Metabolism. 1981;**52**:252-255

[3] Kuhl H. Pharmacology of estrogens and progestogens: Influence of different routes of administration. Climacteric. 2005;**8**(Suppl. 1):3-63

[4] Martínez VF, Ramírez I, Pérez-Campos E, Latorre K, Lete I. Venous and pulmonary thromboembolism and combined hormonal contraceptives. Systematic review and meta-analysis. The European Journal of Contraception & Reproductive Health Care. 2012;**17**(1): 7-29

[5] Paris F, Balaguer P, Rimbault F, Gaspari L, Sultan C. Molecular action of norgestimate: New developments. Gynecological Endocrinology. 2015; **31**(6):487-490

[6] Kuhnz W, Blade H, Mahler M. Systemic availability of levonorgestrel after single oral administration of a norgestimate-containing combination oral contraceptive to 12 young women. Contraception. 1994;**49**(3): 255-263

[7] Kuhl H. Comparative pharmacology of newer progestins. Drugs. 1996;**51**: 188-215

[8] Moore AM, Coolen LM, Porter DT, et al. KNDy cells revisited. Endocrinology. 2018;**159**(9):3219-3234

[9] Fedotcheva TA, Fedotcheva NI, Shimanovsky NL. Progesterone as an anti-inflammatory drug and Immunomodulator: New aspects in hormonal regulation of the inflammation. Biomolecules. 2022;**12**: 1299

[10] Maeda N, Izumiya C, Taniguchi K, et al. Dienogest improves human leucocyte antigen-DR under-expression and reduces tumour necrosis factor-α production in peritoneal fluid cells from women with endometriosis. European Journal of Obstetrics, Gynecology, and Reproductive Biology. 2014;**177**:48-51

[11] Timmer CJ, Geurts TB. Bioequivalence assessment of three different estradiol formulations in postmenopausal women in an open, randomized, single-dose, 3-way cross-over study. European Journal of Drug Metabolism and Pharmacokinetics. 1999; **24**(1):47-53

[12] Stanczyk FZ, Archer DF, Bhavnani BR. Ethinyl estradiol and 17β-estradiol in combined oral contraceptives: Pharmacokinetics, pharmacodynamics and risk assessment. Contraception. 2013 Jun; **87**(6):706-727

[13] Duijkers IJM, Klipping C, Zimmerman Y, Appels N, et al. Inhibition of ovulation by administration of estetrol in combination with drospirenone or levonorgestrel: Results of a phase II dose-finding pilot study. The European Journal of Contraception & Reproductive Health Care. 2015; **20**(6):476-489

[14] Benoit T, Valera MC, Fontaine C, Buscato M, et al. Estetrol, a Fetal selective Estrogen receptor modulator,

acts on the vagina of mice through nuclear Estrogen receptor α activation. The American Journal of Pathology. 2017;**187**(11):2499-2507

[15] Abot A, Fontaine C, Buscato M, Solinhac R. The uterine and vascular actions of estetrol delineate a distinctive profile of estrogen receptor α modulation, uncoupling nuclear and membrane activation. EMBO Molecular Medicine. 2014;**6**(10):1328-1346

[16] Holinka CF, Diczfalusy E, Coelingh Bennink HJ. Estetrol: A unique steroid in human pregnancy. Journal of Steroid Biochemistry & Molecular Biology. 2008;**110**:138-143

[17] Coelingh Bennink HJT, Singer C, Simoncini T, et al. Estetrol, a pregnancy-specific human steroid, prevents and suppresses mammary tumor growth in a rat model. Climacteric. 2008;**11**(Suppl. 1):29

[18] Pluchino N, Santoro AN, Casarosa E, Giannini A, et al. Effect of estetrol administration on brain and serum allopregnanolone in intact and ovariectomized rats. The Journal of Steroid Biochemistry and Molecular Biology. 2014;**143**:285-290

[19] Tskitishvili E, Pequeux C, Munaut C, Viellevoye R, et al. Estrogen receptors and estetrol-dependent neuroprotective actions: A pilot study. The Journal of Endocrinology. 2017;**232**(1):85-95

[20] Endrikat J, Parke S, Trummer D, Serrani M, et al. Pituitary, ovarian and additional contraceptive effects of an estradiol-based combined oral contraceptive: Results of a randomized, open-label study. Contraception. 2013; **87**(2):227-234

[21] Christin-Maitre S, Laroche E, Bricaire L. A new contraceptive pill containing 17β-estradiol and nomegestrol acetate. Womens Health (Lond). 2013;**9**(1):13-23

[22] Klipping C, Duijkers I, Mawet M, Maillard C, et al. Endocrine and metabolic effects of an oral contraceptive containing estetrol and drospirenone. Contraception. 2021; **103**(4):213-221

[23] Stanczyk FZ. Pharmacokinetics and potency of progestins used for hormone replacement therapy and contraception. Reviews in Endocrine & Metabolic Disorders. 2002;**3**(3):211-224

[24] Sasagawa S, Shimizu Y, Imada K, Mizuguchi K. Pharmacological and clinical profile of dienogest. Nihon Yakurigaku Zasshi. 2009;**133**(1):32-40

[25] Shimizu Y, Mita S, Takeuchi T, Notsu T, et al. Dienogest, a synthetic progestin, inhibits prostaglandin E2 production and aromatase expression by human endometrial epithelial cells in a spheroid culture system. Steroids. 2011; **76**(1–2):60-67

[26] Yamanaka K, Xu B, Suganuma I, Kusuki I, et al. Dienogest inhibits aromatase and cyclooxygenase-2 expression and prostaglandin E_2 production in human endometriotic stromal cells in spheroid culture. Fertility and Sterility. 2012;**97**(2):477-482

[27] Miyashita M, Koga K, Takamura M, Izumi G, et al. Dienogest reduces proliferation, aromatase expression and angiogenesis, and increases apoptosis in human endometriosis. Gynecological Endocrinology. 2014; **30**(9):644-648

[28] Lello S. Nomegestrol acetate: Pharmacology, safety profile and therapeutic efficacy. Drugs. 2010;**70**: 541-559

[29] Ruan X, Seeger H, Mueck AO. The pharmacology of nomegestrol acetate. Maturitas. 2012;**71**(4): 345-353

[30] Jaisser F, Farman N. Emerging roles of the mineralocorticoid receptor in pathology: Toward new paradigms in clinical pharmacology. Pharmacological Reviews. 2016;**68**:49-75

[31] Armani A, Cinti F, Marzolla V, Morgan J, et al. Mineralocorticoid receptor antagonism induces browning of white adipose tissue through impairment of autophagy and prevents adipocyte dysfunction in high-fat-diet-fed mice. The FASEB Journal. 2014; **28**(8):3745-3757

[32] Genazzani AR, Pluchino N, Begliuomini S, Pieri M, et al. Drospirenone increases central and peripheral beta-endorphin in ovariectomized female rats. Menopause. 2007;**14**(1):63-73

[33] Makabe T, Koga K, Miyashita M, Takeuchi A, et al. Drospirenone reduces inflammatory cytokines, vascular endothelial growth factor (VEGF) and nerve growth factor (NGF) expression in human endometriotic stromal cells. Journal of Reproductive Immunology. 2017;**119**:44-48

[34] Archer DF, Mansour D, Foidart JM. Bleeding patterns of Oral contraceptives with a cyclic dosing regimen: An overview. Journal of Clinical Medicine. 2022;**11**:4634

[35] Gemzell-Danielsson K, Apter D, Zatik J, Weyers S, et al. Estetrol-Drospirenone combination oral contraceptive: A clinical study of contraceptive efficacy, bleeding pattern and safety in Europe and Russia. BJOG. 2022;**29**(1):63-71

[36] Ahrendt HJ, Makalová D, Parke S, Mellinger U, Diana MD. Bleeding pattern and cycle control with an estradiol-based oral contraceptive: A seven-cycle, randomized comparative trial of estradiol valerate/dienogest and ethinyl estradiol/levonorgestre. Contraception. 2009;**80**(5):436-444

[37] Nelson A, Parke S, Mellinger U, Zampaglione E, Schmidt A. Efficacy and safety of a combined oral contraceptive containing estradiol valerate/dienogest: Results from a clinical study conducted in North America. Journal of Women's Health (Larchmt). Mar 2014;**23**(3): 204-210

[38] Jensen JT, Bitzer J, Nappi RE, Ahlers C. Pooled analysis of bleeding profile, efficacy and safety of oral oestradiol valerate/dienogest in women aged 25 and under. The European Journal of Contraception & Reproductive Health Care. 2020;**25**(2):98-105

[39] Mansour D, Westhoff C, Kher U, Korver T. Pooled analysis of two randomized, open-label studies comparing the effects of nomegestrol acetate/17β-estradiol and drospirenone/ethinyl estradiol on bleeding patterns in healthy women. Contraception. 2017; **95**(4):390-397

[40] Bitzer J, Parke S, Roemer T, Serrani M. Endometrial safety of an oral contraceptive containing estradiol valerate and dienogest. International Journal of Women's Health. 2011;**3**: 127-132

[41] Duijkers I, Klipping C, Kinet V, Jost M, et al. Effects of an oral contraceptive containing estetrol and drospirenone on ovarian function. Contraception. 2021;**103**(6):386-393

[42] Elmaoğulları S, Ayca Z. Abnormal uterine bleeding in adolescents. Journal

of Clinical Research in Pediatric Endocrinology. 2018;**10**(3):191-197

[43] Nichols WL, Hultin MB, James AH, et al. von Willebrand disease (VWD): Evidence-based diagnosis and management guidelines, the National Heart, Lung, and Blood Institute (NHLBI) expert panel report (USA). Haemophilia. 2008;**14**(2):171-232

[44] Nelson JM, Compton SD, Farahzad MM, Winfrey OK, Rosen MW. The relationship between estrogen and subsequent growth restriction among adolescents with heavy menstrual bleeding at menarche. Journal of Pediatric Endocrinology & Metabolism. 2023;**36**(3):255-260

[45] Bahamondes L, Valeria Bahamondes M, Shulman LP. Non-contraceptive benefits of hormonal and intrauterine reversible contraceptive methods. Human Reproduction Update. 2015;**21**(5):640-651

[46] Lethaby A, Wise MR, Weterings MA, Bofill Rodriguez M, Brown J. Combined hormonal contraceptives for heavy menstrual bleeding. Cochrane Database of Systematic Reviews. 2019;**2**(2):CD00015

[47] Jensen JT. Evaluation of a new estradiol oral contraceptive: Estradiol valerate and dienogest. Expert Opinion on Pharmacotherapy. 2010;**11**(7): 1147-1157

[48] Fraser IS, Römer T, Parke S, Zeun S, et al. Effective treatment of heavy and/or prolonged menstrual bleeding with an oral contraceptive containing estradiol valerate and dienogest: A randomized, double-blind phase III trial. Human Reproduction. 2011;**26**(10):2698-2708

[49] Rafie S, Borgelt L, Koepf ER, Temple-Cooper ME, et al. Novel oral contraceptive for heavy menstrual bleeding: Estradiol valerate and dienogest. International Journal of Women's Health. 2013;**5**:313-321

[50] Weisberg E, Mc Geehan K, Hangan G, Fraser IS. Potentially effective therapy of heavy menstrual bleeding with an oestradiol-nomegestrole acetate contraceptive: A pilot study. Pilot and Feasibility Studies. 2017;**3**:18-25

[51] Marquardt RM, Tim TH, Shin Y, Jeong J. Progesterone and estrogen signaling in the endometrium: What goes wrong in endometriosis? International Journal of Molecular Sciences. 2019;**20**: 3822

[52] Dunselman GAJ, Vermeulen N, Becker C, et al. European Society of Human Reproduction and Embryology ESHRE guideline: Management of women with endometriosis. Human Reproduction. Mar 2014;**29**(3):400-412

[53] Somigliana E, Viganò P, La Sala GB, Balasini M, et al. Follicular fluid as a favourable environment for endometrial and endometriotic cell growth in vitro. Human Reproduction. 2001;**16**(6): 1076-1078

[54] Dinh A, Sriprasert I, Williams AR, Archer DF. A review of the endometrial histologic effects of progestins and progesterone receptors modulators in reproductive age women. Contraception. 2015;**91**:360-367

[55] Mabrouk M, Solfrini S, Frascà C, Del Forno S, et al. A new oral contraceptive regimen for endometriosis management: Preliminary experience with 24/4-day drospirenone/ethinylestradiol 3 mg/20 mcg. Gynecological Endocrinology. 2012;**28**(6):451-454

[56] Yoshino O, Suzukamo Y, Yoshihara K, Takahash N. Quality of life

in Japanese patients with dysmenorrhea or endometriosis-associated pelvic pain treated with extended regimen Ethinylestradiol/Drospirenone in a real-world setting: A prospective observational study. Advances in Therapy. 2022;**39**:5087-5104

[57] Caruso S, Iraci M, Cianci S, Fava V, et al. Comparative, open-label prospective study on the quality of life and sexual function of women affected by endometriosis-associated pelvic pain on 2 mg dienogest/30 μg ethinyl estradiol continuous or 21/7 regimen oral contraceptive. Journal of Endocrinological Investigation. 2016; **39**(8):923-931

[58] Vercellini P, Barbara G, Somigliana E, Bianchi S, et al. Comparison of contraceptive ring and patch for the treatment of symptomatic endometriosis. Fertility and Sterility. 2010;**93**:2150-2161

[59] Priya K, Rajaram S, Goel N. Comparison of combined hormonal vaginal ring and low dose combined oral hormonal pill for the treatment of idiopathic chronic pelvic pain: A randomised trial. European Journal of Obstetrics, Gynecology, and Reproductive Biology. 2016;**207**:141-146

[60] Becker CM, Gattrell WT, Gude K, Singh SS. Reevaluating response and failure of medical treatment of endometriosis: A systematic review. Fertility and Sterility. 2017;**108**(1): 125-136

[61] Vercellini P, Buggio L, Berlanda N, Barbara G, et al. Estrogen-progestins and progestins for the management of endometriosis. Fertility and Sterility. 2016;**106**:1552-1571

[62] Alcalde AM, Martínez-Zamora MA, Gracia M, Ros C, et al. Assessment of quality of life, sexual quality of life, and pain symptoms in deep infiltrating endometriosis patients with or without associated Adenomyosis and the influence of a flexible extended combined Oral contraceptive regimen: Results of a prospective, observational study. The Journal of Sexual Medicine. 2022;**19**(2):311-318

[63] Vercellini P, Buggio L, Frattaruolo MP, Borghi A, et al. Medical treatment of endometriosis-related pain. Best Practice & Research. Clinical Obstetrics & Gynaecology. 2018;**51**: 68-91

[64] Grandi G, Xholli A, Napolitano A, Palma F, Cagnacci A. Pelvic pain and quality of life of women with endometriosis during quadriphasic estradiol valerate/dienogest oral contraceptive: A patient-preference prospective 24-week pilot study. Reproductive Sciences. 2015;**22**(5): 626-632

[65] Mariani LL, Novara L, Mancarella M, Fuso L, et al. Estradiol/nomegestrol acetate as a first-line and rescue therapy for the treatment of ovarian and deep infiltrating endometriosis. Gynecological Endocrinology. 2021;**37**(7):646-649

[66] Caruso S, Cianci A, Iraci M, Fava V, et al. Does Nomegestrol acetate plus 17β-Estradiol Oral contraceptive improve endometriosis-associated chronic pelvic pain in women? Journal of Women's Health (2002). 2020;**29**(9):1184-1191

[67] Patiño-García D, Palomino J, Pomés C, Celle C, et al. Estetrol increases progesterone genetic response without triggering common estrogenic effects in Endometriotic cell lines and primary cultures. Biomedicine. 2023;**11**(4):1169

[68] Harada T, Kosaka S, Elliesen J, Yasuda M, et al. Ethinylestradiol 20 μg/

drospirenone 3 mg in a flexible extended regimen for the management of endometriosis-associated pelvic pain: A randomized controlled trial. Fertility and Sterility. 2017;**108**(5):798-805

[69] El Taha L, Abu Musa A, Khalifeh D, Khalil A, Abbasi S, Nassif J. Efficacy of dienogest vs combined oral contraceptive on pain associated with endometriosis: Randomized clinical trial. European Journal of Obstetrics, Gynecology, and Reproductive Biology. 2021;**267**:205-212

[70] Piacenti I, Viscardi MF, Masciullo L, Sangiuliano C, Scaramuzzino S, et al. Dienogest versus continuous oral levonorgestrel/EE in patients with endometriosis: what's the best choice? Gynecological Endocrinology. 2021; **37**(5):471-475

[71] Angioni S, Pontis A, Malune ME, Cela V, et al. Is dienogest the best medical treatment for ovarian endometriomas? Results of a multicentric case control study. Gynecological Endocrinology. 2020; **36**(1):84-86

[72] Maiorana A, Alfano P, Mercurio A, Marcantonio S, et al. Quality of life and clinical factors in women with endometriosis, the role of dienogest vs EE/dienogest over time: A single-center study. Archiv Gynecol Obstet. 2023;**307**: 1503-1512

[73] Caruso S, Cianci A, Sareri MI, Panella M, et al. Randomized study on the efectiveness of nomegestrol acetate plus 17β-estradiol oral contraceptive versus dienogest oral pill in women with suspected endometriosis-associated chronic pelvic pain. BMC Women's Health. 2022;**22**:146

[74] Mehdizadeh Kashi A, Niakan G, Ebrahimpour M, et al. A randomized, double-blind, placebo-controlled pilot study of the comparative effects of dienogest and the combined oral contraceptive pill in women with endometriosis. International Journal of Gynecology & Obstetrics. 2021;**00**:1-9

[75] Granese R, Perino A, Calagna G, Saitta S, et al. Gonadotrophin-releasing hormone analogue or dienogest plus estradiol valerate to prevent pain recurrence after laparoscopic surgery for endometriosis: A multi-center randomized trial. Acta Obstetricia et Gynecologica Scandinavica. 2015;**94**(6): 637-645

[76] Wattanayingcharoenchai R, Rattanasiri S, Charakorn C, Attia J, et al. Post-operative hormonal treatment for prevention of endometrioma recurrence after ovarian cystectomy: A systematic review and network meta-analysis. BJOG. 2021;**128**(1):25-35

[77] Zakhari A, Delpero E, McKeown S, Tomlinson G, ct al. Endometriosis recurrence following post-operative hormonal suppression: A systematic review and meta-analysis. Human Reproduction Update. 2021;**27**(1):96-107

[78] Vannuccini S, Lazzeri L, Orlandini C, Morgante G, et al. Mental health, pain symptoms and systemic comorbidities in women with endometriosis: A cross-sectional study. Journal of Psychosomatic Obstetrics and Gynaecology. 2018;**39**(4):315-320

[79] Gambadauro P, Carli V, Hadlaczky G. Depressive symptoms among women with endometriosis: A systematic review and meta-analysis. American Journal of Obstetrics and Gynecology. 2019;**220**(3):230-241

[80] van Barneveld E, Manders J, van Osch FMH, van Poll M, et al. Depression,

anxiety, and correlating factors in endometriosis: A systematic review and meta-analysis. Journal of Women's Health (2002). 2022;**31**(2):219-230

[81] McCloskey LR, Wisner KL, Cattan MK, Betcher HK. Contraception for women with psychiatric disorders. The American Journal of Psychiatry. 2021;**178**(3):247-255

[82] Borgström A, Odlind V, Ekselius L, Sundström-Poromaa I. Adverse mood effects of combined oral contraceptives in relation to personality traits. European Journal of Obstetrics, Gynecology, and Reproductive Biology. 2008;**141**(2): 127-130

[83] Skovlund CW, Mørch LS, Kessing LV, Lidegaard O. Association of Hormonal Contraception with depression. JAMA Psychiatry. 2016; **73**(11):1154-1162

[84] Zettermark S, Perez Vicente R, Merlo J. Hormonal contraception increases the risk of psychotropic drug use in adolescent girls but not in adults: A pharmaco-epidemiological study on 800 000 Swedish women. PLoS One. 2018;**13**(3):e0194773

[85] de Wit AE, Booij SH, Giltay EJ, Joffe H, et al. Association of use of Oral contraceptives with depressive symptoms among adolescents and Young women. JAMA Psychiatry. 2020; **77**(1):52-59

[86] Schaffir J, Worly BL, Gur TL. Combined hormonal contraception and its effects on mood: A critical review. The European Journal of Contraception & Reproductive Health Care. 2016;**21**(5): 347-355

[87] Pagano HP, Zapata LB, Berry-Bibee EN, Nanda K, et al. Safety of hormonal contraception and intrauterine devices among women with depressive and bipolar disorders: A systematic review. Contraception. 2016;**94**(6):641-649

[88] McKetta S, Keyes KM. Oral contraceptive use and depression among adolescents. Annals of Epidemiology. 2019;**29**:46-51

[89] Robakis T, Williams KE, Nutkiewicz L, Rasgon NL. Hormonal contraceptives and mood: Review of the literature and implications for future research. Current Psychiatry Reports. 2019;**21**(7):57

[90] Young EA, Kornstein SG, Harvey AT, Wisniewski SR, et al. Influences of hormone-based contraception on depressive symptoms in premenopausal women with major depression. Psychoneuroendocrinology. 2007;**32**(7):843-853

[91] Toffol E, Heikinheimo O, Koponen P, Luoto R, et al. Hormonal contraception and mental health: Results of a population-based study. Human Reproduction. 2011;**26**(11):3085-3093

[92] Jenabi E, Khazaei S. Endometriosis and migraine headache risk: A meta-analysis. Women & Health. 2020;**60**(8): 939-945

[93] Wu Y, Wang H, Chen S, Lin Y, et al. Migraine is more prevalent in advanced-stage endometriosis, especially when co-occuring with Adenomoysis. Frontiers in Endocrinology (Lausanne). 2022;**12**: 814474

[94] Miller JA, Missmer SA, Vitonis AF, et al. Prevalence of migraines in adolescents with endometriosis. Fertility and Sterility. 2018;**109**(4):685-690

[95] Maia H Jr, Casoy T, Correia T, Freitas L, et al. Effect of the menstrual

cycle and oral contraceptives on aromatase and cyclooxygenase-2 expression in adenomyosis. Gynecological Endocrinology. 2006; **22**(10):547-555

[96] Vannuccini S, Luisi S, Tosti C, Sorbi F, et al. Role of medical therapy in the management of uterine adenomyosis. Fertility and Sterility. 2018;**109**(3):398-405

[97] Naftalin J, Hoo W, Pateman K, Mavrelos D, et al. Is adenomyosis associated with menorrhagia? Human Reproduction. 2014;**29**(3):473-479

[98] Benetti-Pinto CL, Mira TAA, Yela DA, Teatin-Juliato CR, et al. Pharmacological treatment for symptomatic Adenomyosis: A systematic review. Revista Brasileira de Ginecologia e Obstetrícia. 2019;**41**(9):564-574

[99] Cope AG, Ainsworth AJ, Stewart EA. Current and future medical therapies for Adenomyosis. Seminars in Reproductive Medicine. 2020;**38**(2–03):151-156

[100] Zimmerman Y, Eijkemans MJC, Coelingh Bennink HJT, Blankenstein MA, et al. The effect of combined oral contraception on testosterone levels in healthy women: A systematic review and meta-analysis. Human Reproduction Update. 2014; **20**(1):76-105

[101] Mawet M, Maillard C, Klipping C, Zimmerman Y, et al. Unique effects on hepatic function, lipid metabolism, bone and growth endocrine parameters of estetrol in combined oral contraceptives. The European Journal of Contraception & Reproductive Health Care. 2015;**20**: 463-475

[102] Teede HJ, Misso ML, Costello MF, Dokras A, et al. Recommendations from the international evidence-based guideline for the assessment and management of polycystic ovary syndrome. Human Reproduction. 2018; **33**(9):1602-1618

[103] Rabe T, Kowald A, Ortmann J, Rehberger-Schneider S. Inhibition of skin 5 alpha-reductase by oralcontraceptive progestins in vitro. Gynecological Endocrinology. 2000; **14**(4):223-230

[104] Carmina E, Dreno B, Lucky WA, Agak WG, et al. Female adult acne and androgen excess: A report from the multidisciplinary androgen excess and PCOS committee. Journal of the Endocrine Society. 2022;**6**(3):bvac003

[105] Ju Q, Tao T, Hu T, Serap Karadağ A, et al. Sex hormones and acne. Clinics in Dermatology. 2017;**35**(2): 130-137

[106] Cibula D, Fanta M, Vrbikova J, Stanicka S, et al. The effect of combination therapy with metformin and combined oral contraceptives (COC) versus COC alone on insulin sensitivity, hyperandrogenaemia, SHBG and lipids in PCOS patients. Human Reproduction. 2005;**20**(1):180-184

[107] Di Carlo C, Gargano V, Sparice S, Tommaselli GA, et al. Effects of an oral contraceptive containing estradiol valerate and dienogest on circulating androgen levels and acne in young patients with PCOS: An observational preliminary study. Gynecological Endocrinology. 2013;**29**(12):1048-1050

[108] Teede HJ, Misso ML, Costello MF, Dokras A, et al. International PCOS network. Recommendations from the international evidence-based guideline for the assessment and management of polycystic ovary syndrome. Fertility and Sterility. 2018;**110**(3):364-379

[109] Goodman NF, Cobin RH, Futterweit W, Glueck JS, et al. American Association of Clinical Endocrinologists (AACE); American College of Endocrinology (ACE); androgen excess and PCOS society guide to the best practices in the evaluation and treatment of polycystic ovary syndrome -part 1. Endocrine Practice. 2015;**21**(12): 1415-1426

[110] Falsetti L, Gambera A, Platto C, Legrenzi L. Management of hirsutism. American Journal of Clinical Dermatology. 2000;**1**(2):89-99

[111] Plu-Bureau G, Maitrot-Mantelet L, Hugon-Rodin J, Canonico M. Hormonal contraceptives and venous thromboembolism: An epidemiological update. Best Practice & Research. Clinical Endocrinology & Metabolism. 2013;**27**(1):25-34

[112] de Bastos M, Stegeman BH, Rosendaal FR, Van Hylckama Vlieg A, et al. Combined oral contraceptives: Venous thrombosis. Cochrane Database of Systematic Reviews. 2014;**3**(3): CD010813

[113] Hugon-Rodin J, Gompel A, Plu-Bureau G. Epidemiology of hormonal contraceptives related venous thromboembolism. European Journal of Endocrinology. 2014;**171**:R221-RR23

[114] Vinogradova Y, Coupland C, Hippisley-Cox J. Use of combined oral contraceptives and risk of venous thromboembolism: Nested case-control studies using the QResearch and CPRD databases. BMJ. 2015;**350**:h2135

[115] Dragoman MV, Tepper NK, Fu R, Curtis KM, et al. A systematic review and meta-analysis of venous thrombosis risk among users of combined oral contraception. International Journal of Gynaecology and Obstetrics. 2018; **141**(3):287-229

[116] Dinger J, Monher S, Heinemann K. Combined oral contraceptives containing dienogest and estradiol valerate may carry a lower risk of venous and arterial thromboembolism compared to conventional preparations: Results from the extended INAS-SCORE study. Front Womens Health. 2020;**5**:1-8

[117] Reed S, Koro C, DiBello J, Becker K, et al. Prospective controlled cohort study on the safety of a monophasic oral contraceptive containing nomegestrol acetate (2.5mg) and 17β-oestradiol (1.5mg) (PRO-E2 study): Risk of venous and arterial thromboembolism. The European Journal of Contraception & Reproductive Health Care. 2021;**26**(6): 439-446

Section 3

Non-Hormonal Contraceptions Methods

Chapter 5

Advances in Hormone-Free Contraceptive Devices

Alfred A. Shihata, Steven A. Brody and Birgit Linderoth

Abstract

Up to (99%) of women worldwide may use birth control for at least 30 years. However, most modern female contraceptives containing hormones can have undesirable side effects. Among the limited hormone-free options, the fertility awareness method is the safest and most effective when used correctly. This study explores a time-tested, safe, and effective barrier contraceptive called FemCap. FemCap not only aids in pinpointing the day of ovulation but also integrates electronic period-tracking technology to enhance the efficacy of the fertility awareness method. Stress Urinary Incontinence is a prevalent issue affecting women of all ages, often suffering in silence. Our research aims to address the unmet needs in women's reproductive health. We have discovered that FemCap can function as a pessary to manage Stress Urinary Incontinence by providing support to the bladder neck and straightening the urethra, thereby restoring the competence of the urethral sphincters. FemCap has emerged as a powerhouse for fertility awareness and stress urinary incontinence. However, due to the limitations of this study, the authors welcome any investigators who can validate our findings as well as provide suggestions to enhance the overall value of this research for the benefit of all women.

Keywords: hormone-free barrier contraception, fertility awareness methods, FemCap, stress urinary incontinence, vaginal drug delivery, pairing FemCap with electronic period tracking application

1. Introduction

The authors organized a series of small focus groups to discover what women consider the ideal birth control (**Figure 1**). Over the past decade, a noteworthy breakthrough has been the creation of a hormone-free contraceptive device known as Caya diaphragm, which is designed to fit most women due to its unique one-size feature (**Figure 2**). Microbicides are experimental products that could prevent Human Immune Virus (HIV) transmission from male to female and vice versa (**Figure 3**).

Male and Female condoms are the only devices approved for preventing Sexually transmitted diseases (STDs). Though FemCap is not approved for the prevention of STIs, it has all the biological and plausible potential for the prevention of STIs, see the comparative (**Table 1**).

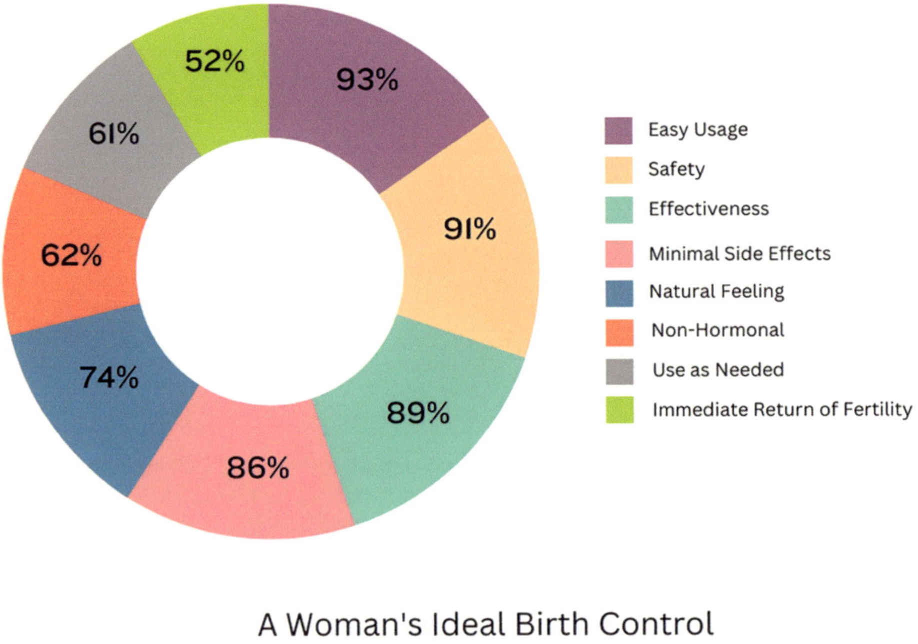

Figure 1.
A women's ideal birth control.

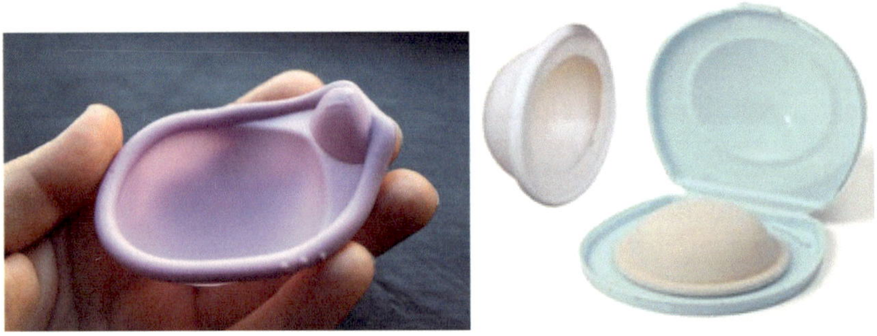

Figure 2.
Caya Diaphragm vs. Wide Seal Diaphragm.

2. FemCap design and its evolution

The cervix was determined to be the main portal of entry for HIV and Sexual Transmitted Infections (STI) organisms for transmission from men to women. This is due to the Os opening of the cervix as well as the presence of chemokine co-receptors for HIV on the cervix, called Chemo Chine Receptor 5 (CCR5) and Chemo X Receptor 4 (CXR4). HIV first fuses with these co-receptors and then invades the immune cell CD4 (**Figure 4**) [1].

In response to the HIV/Acquired Immune Deficiency Syndrome (AIDS) pandemic and according to the scientific recommendation for the prevention of transmission of HIV from male to female [2], the first author developed the

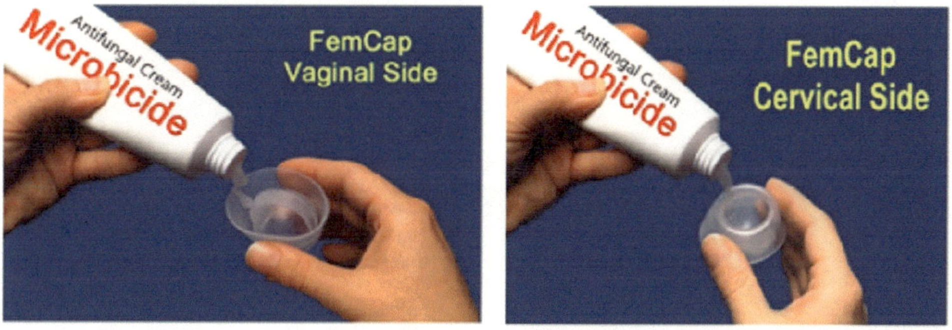

Figure 3.
FemCap Used to Deliver Microbicide.

FemCap, specifically designed to mechanically covers and seal the cervix and store and deliver the microbicide. He also developed a microbicide/spermicide to kill the sperm and invading HIV and STIs organisms upon deposition into the vagina. Both were patented [3, 4]. However, the microbicide was abandoned due to the presence of Nonoxyle-9.

Comparison of the Male and Female Condoms with the FemCap

	Male Condom	**Female Condom**	**The FemCap**
Gender Control	Male – controlled	Female- Controlled	100% percent woman-controlled and can be applied without the knowledge of the man.
Spontaneity of intercourse	The condom interrupts the spontaneity of intercourse to both partners, which may lead to inconsistent use.	Can be applied 8 hours in advance of intercourse.	The FemCap does not interrupt spontaneity as it should be applied before sexual arousal.
Sexual sensations	It reduces the pleasurable sensation of intercourse to both partners.	Impaired sensation to both Male and Female	It does not reduce sensation to either partner.
Acceptability	It is not accepted by either partner, particularly the male	It is NOT Accepted by both partners. Particularly the female. It may not be used at all	It is well accepted by both partners
User failure	Men must apply the condom on erect penis. They must rush to avoid the loss of erection. This may lead to incorrect application or skipping the application completely.	User failure is common. Males penetrate between the condom and vagina, Condom expelled before, or during intercourse, which lead to failure.	The FemCap must be applied before any sexual arousal when the woman is not rushed. Once the woman learns how to apply the Fem Cap it will become an easy routine with minimal chance for user's failure.

Comparison of the Male and Female Condoms with the FemCap			
	Male Condom	**Female Condom**	**The FemCap**
Leaking and Breakage	The condom may leak or break even when it is used properly	It may leak	The FemCap does not to leak or break during usual use.
Allergy	Most male condoms are made of Latex, which can cause serious allergic reaction.	It is made of hypoallergenic materials.	Is made of an inert non-allergenic silicone material.
Storage and shelf life	Latex material deteriorates very quickly if it is not stored properly particularly in hot tropical countries.	Storage at room temperature Has longer shelf life	Is made of durable material that can withstand extreme temperatures without any deterioration.
Cost	Costs $.90 - $1.00 for a single use.	Cost $ 2–4 Dollars for a single use.	It comes with an instructional video online and Costs $89, and it is reusable for 1–2 years, depending on the user.
Typical effectiveness	Effectiveness depends. on the user. 83%	Effectiveness depends on the user. 79%	Effectiveness depends on the user. 92.4%
STIs prevention	If used properly from the beginning to the end of intercourse.	If used properly from the beginning to the end of intercourse.	Has the plausible potential for, Prevention however, it was not yet tested.
Hazard to environment	May pose environmental hazard if not properly disposed.	May pose environmental hazard if not properly disposed	Does not pose any environmental hazard.

Table 1.
Comparison of the Male and Female Condom with the FemCap.

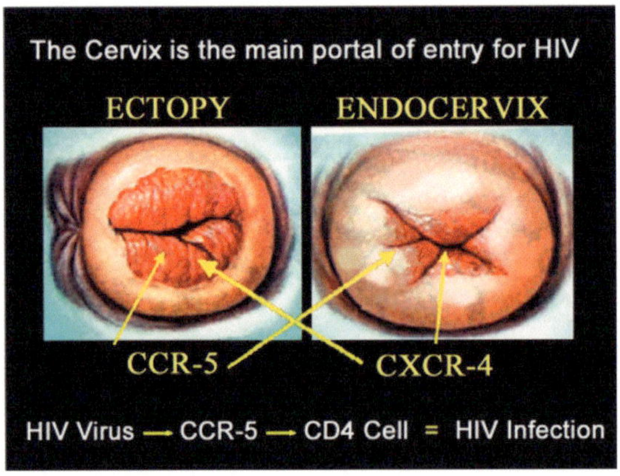

Figure 4.
HIV + CCR5+ CXR4 + CD4 cell = AIDS infection.

DOI: http://dx.doi.org/10.5772/intechopen.112255

The first-generation FemCap (**Figure 5**) was not approved by the Federal Food and Drug Administration (FDA) due to the difficulty of removal and poor efficacy in multiparous women (**Figures 5–10**).

The second generation FemCap that is FDA APPROVED has a removal strap that improved its safety by eliminating the fingernail abrasion to the cervix. The increased dimensions of the brim increased the surface contact between the vagina and the FemCap, improving its stability. This is due to the fact that FemCap is held by the vaginal contraction preventing dislodgment and thus increasing its effectiveness and acceptability.

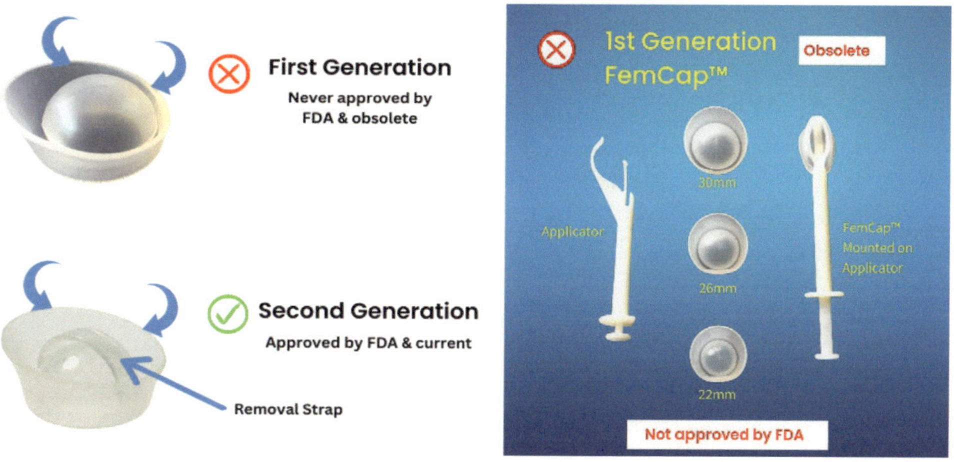

Figure 5.
First generation FemCap and the improved second generation.

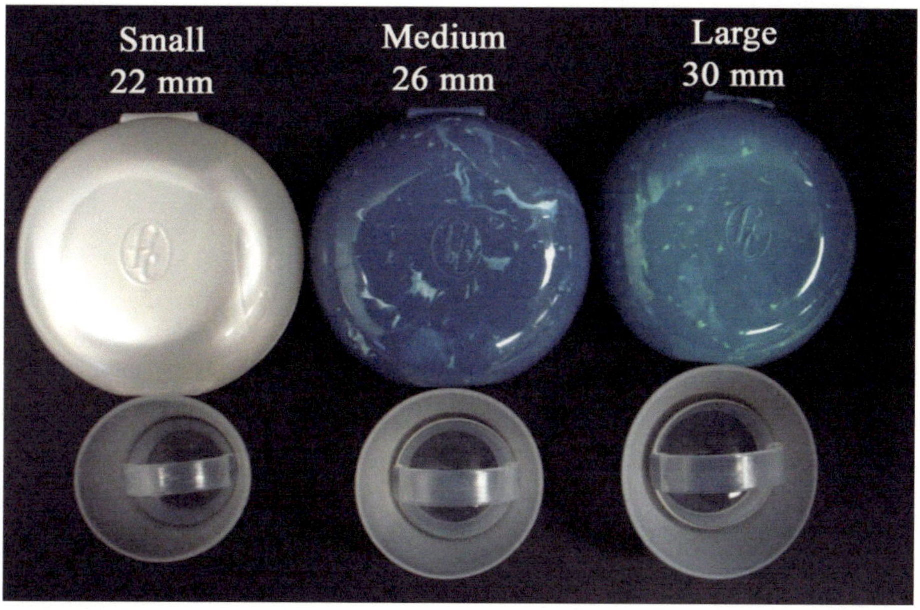

Figure 6.
FemCap three sizes.

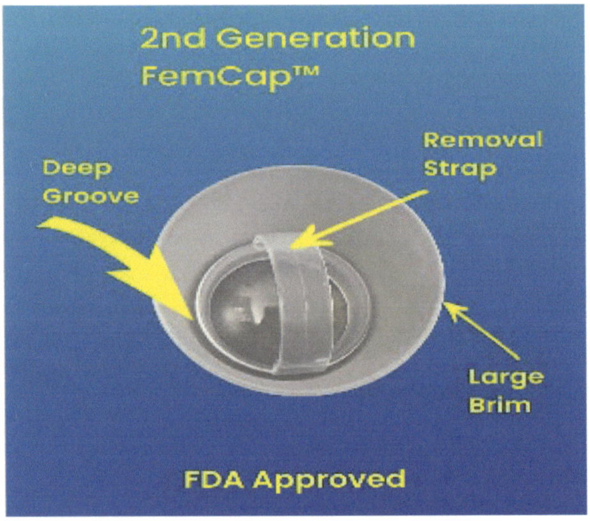

Figure 7.
Second generation showing improvements.

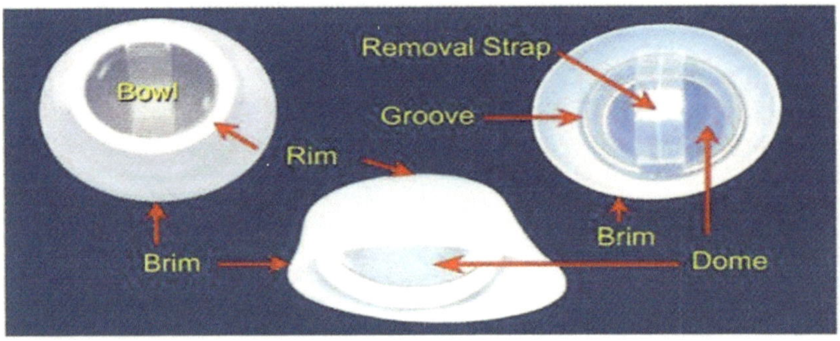

Figure 8.
FemCap diagram all views.

Unfortunately, some institutions still cite the obsolete effective rate of the first generation that was not used or approved by the FDA.

The following Video 1 (https://www.youtube.com/watch?v=4FgvJbl_X_M) will visually demonstrate the difference between the obsolete first-generation and the FDA-APPROVED second-generation. The references [5–8] will cite the difference in the effective rate of the first versus the second-generation FemCap.

Careful consideration was taken when designing FemCap's second-generation model. Its DOME provided full coverage for protecting the cervix and preventing it from prolapsing, while its RIM fits snugly into the vaginal Fornices and encompassed its entrance (**Figures 7–10**). A LIP was implemented to grasp onto her cervix to secure its hold (**Figure 10**). Regarding its BRIM formation, it had an outward flare to press against the inward vaginal contraction (**Figures 7**, **10** and **11**), thus creating a tight seal, preventing sperm from penetrating along the vaginal walls. Anatomically wise as well, it possessed a more extended posterior section than other parts. Together these features bring about a comfortable and secure fitting of the FemCap.

DOI: http://dx.doi.org/10.5772/intechopen.112255

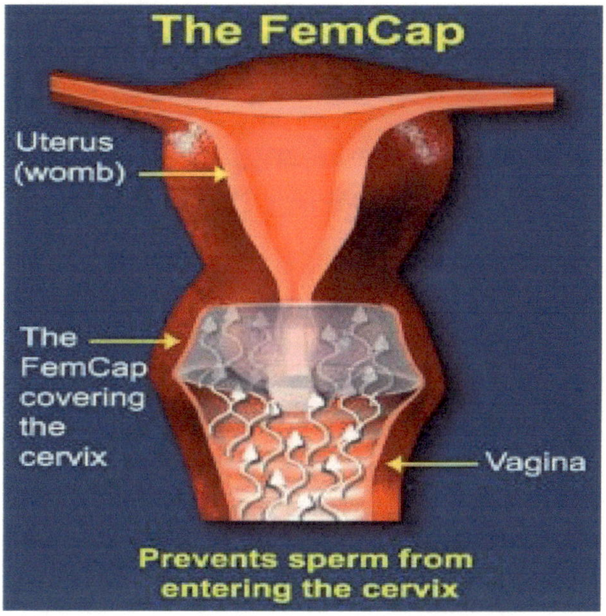

Figure 9.
FemCap covering cervix.

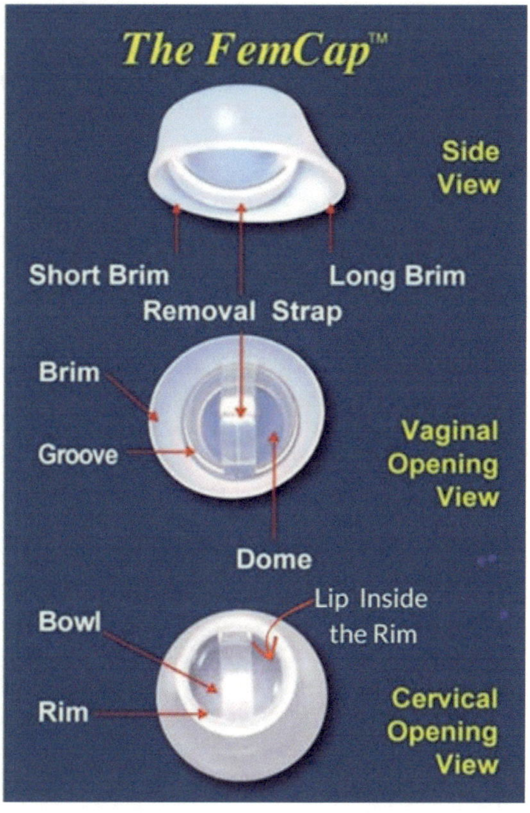

Figure 10.
FemCap views.

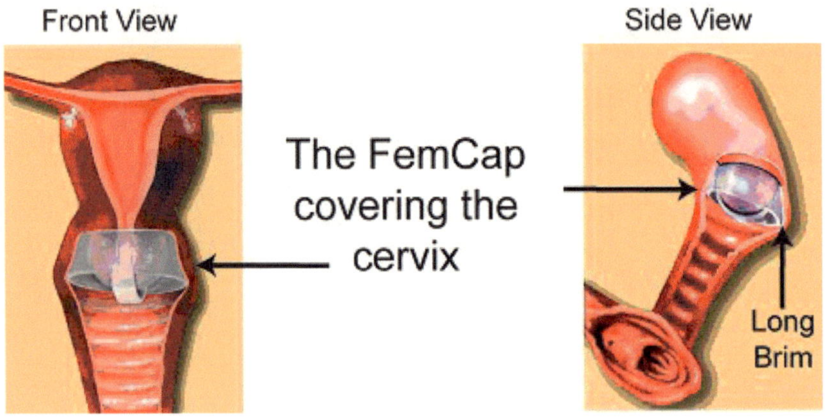

Figure 11.
The FemCap covering the cervix.

3. Size selection

Vaginal anatomy varies in different women and even in the same woman in response to pregnancy and delivery., so a one-size-fits all approach simply will not work. To solve this issue the FemCap comes with three sizes to choose from, the 22 mm for those who have never been pregnant, 26 mm for those who have experienced pregnancy without vaginal delivery (e.g. C-section or miscarriage) and 30 mm for women who have delivered vaginally (**Figure 6**).

Utilizing the 3 sizes eliminated the need for time-consuming and inaccurate measurement and custom fitting. The woman's obstetrical history determines the FemCap size selection.

This study yielded an interesting outcome; the height and weight of women have no or very little relation to cervical diameter or vaginal elasticity. It was found out that pregnancy and delivery are the only factors that influence these two characteristics.

The FemCap is designed with a unique deep groove facing the vaginal opening. (**Figures 6**, 7, and **9**) This groove was intended to trap and expose the sperm and bacteria or viruses to the spermicide upon deposition into the vagina for a prolonged period to ensure the complete killing of sperm and microorganisms (**Figure 7**).

The following Video 2 (https://www.youtube.com/IZkxCbZ0WtU) will visually explain the features of the second Generation FemCap versus the obsolete cervical cap.

FemCap provided a much-needed alternative to traditional hormone-based birth control and was quickly approved for contraception in both United States and Europe. Unfortunately, approval of FemCap for HIV/AIDS prevention was denied due to ethical and logistical considerations (**Figure 12**).

The FemCap is a well-established, time-tested, safe, and effective non-hormonal contraceptive device [5–12]. The FemCap have been used by women world-wide for two decades with good success and without any reported side effects. It has never been withdrawn from any country for any reason. The FemCap's unique storage groove for spermicide/microbicides can potentially be utilized to treat sexually transmitted infections topically (**Figures 8–11**).

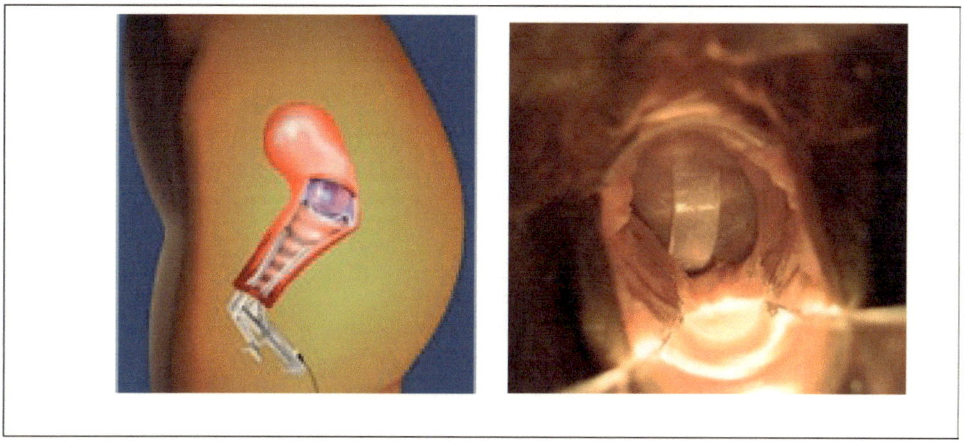

FemCap viewed by Speculum.

Figure 12.
FemCap viewed by speculum.

4. The fertility awareness method

The Fertility Awareness Method (FWM) is the safest and most cost-effective contraceptive method, yet it is the least prescribed by clinicians and used by women. This method does not need equipment, drugs, or professional supervision after the initial training. There is also a common misconception that this method is difficult to learn and has a high failure rate. The subjective observation of collecting the fertile cervical mucous from the underwear or inserting a finger in the vagina may yield a very small amount of cervical secretions mixed with vaginal fluid. All the above factors might lead to missing the fertile window [13, 14].

We spared no effort in enhancing the effectiveness and simplifying the learning of this wonderful method [13–24]. We attributed the high failure rate to the fact that women miss the most vital sign of ovulation and thus miss their fertile window.

We used a two-prong approach to enhance this method's effectiveness and simplify its learning [13–24]. We utilized FemCap to collect the fertile cervical mucous directly from the cervix. Starting 2 days after the end of menstruation until the clear translucent stretchy preovulatory mucous (Spinnbarkeit) (**Figure 13**) appears just before ovulation. The FemCap allowed women to collect a large quantity and excellent quality of their fertile cervical mucous directly from the cervix. The FemCap also prevents the fertile cervical mucous from mixing with other vaginal secretions.

The following Video 3 (https://www.youtube.com/watch?v=oYoYb0gM-w4) will visually teach and simplify the learning of this method.

The second prong was using the Smart Telephone technology (**Figure 14**) to monitor the menstrual cycle and inform women of the fertile and infertile days. This innovative technology allowed women to pinpoint the precise day of ovulation, and thus they can decide whether to become pregnant or prevent it.

We recruited 40 healthy women with regular periods to participate in this pilot research. We randomized twenty women to use the traditional Fertility Awareness Method (FAM) with basal body temperature and the usual subjective

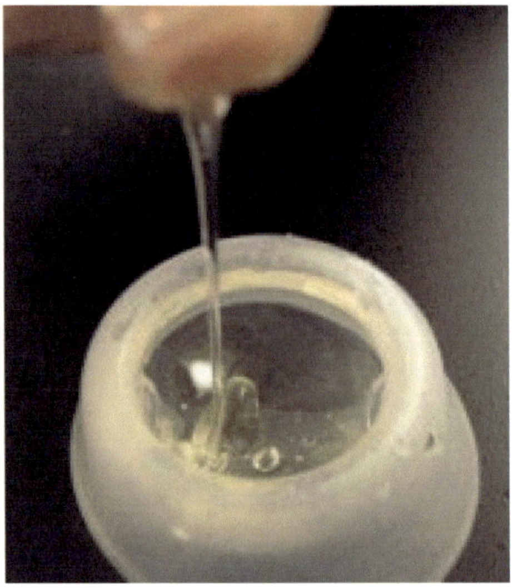

Figure 13.
Spinnbarkeit.

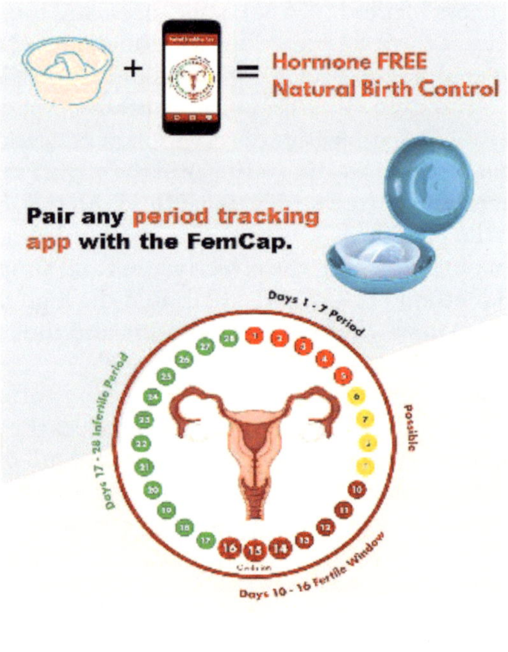

Figure 14.
FemCap paired with period tracking technology.

collection of fertile cervical mucus. The other 20 women used the FemCap to collect their fertile cervical mucus (Spinnbarkeit) directly from the cervix from day nine until they detected fertile mucus [22]. We also instructed women to record their findings and any side effects on the basal temperature chart (**Figure 15**) [14, 23].

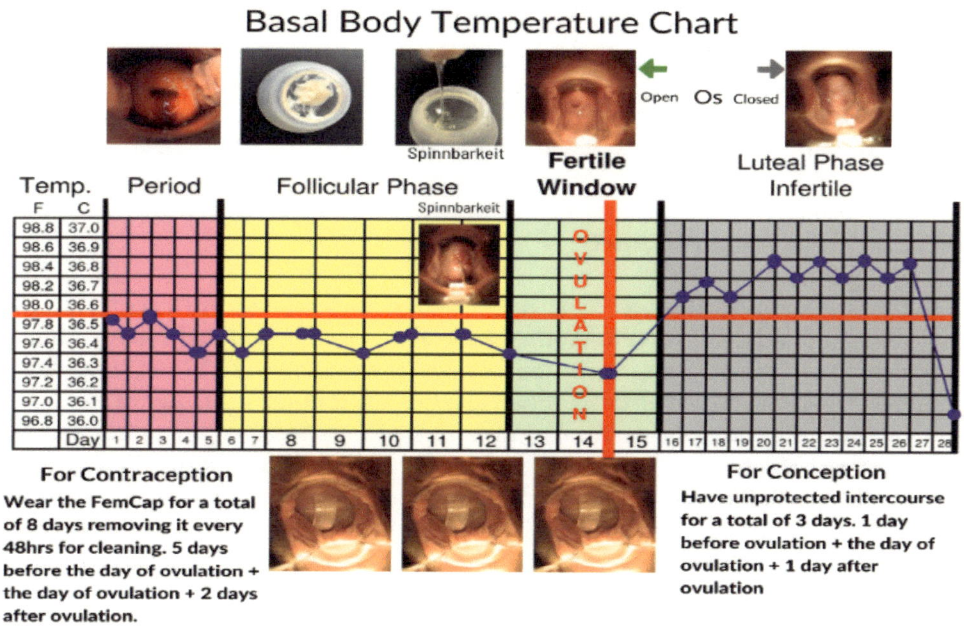

Figure 15.
Basal body temperature chart.

5. Result

The results of this study utilizing the FemCap to collect the cervical mucous showed that 95% of the participants could accurately identify preovulatory fertile cervical mucus. These same users also verified ovulation with a positive urinary L.H. (Luteinizing Hormone) surge, accompanied by biphasic Basal Body Temperature charts (**Figure 15**) that supported the L.H. surge results.

However, the control group that used subjective detection of their fertile cervical mucous were successful in only 55%. Collecting cervical mucus directly from the cervix without mixing with any vaginal fluid content yielded higher quantities and better-quality samples (Spinnbarkeit). This enabled women to shorten fertile window to three days for conception, and eight days for contraception (**Figure 15**).

6. Conclusion

Collecting mucus directly from the cervix yielded a large quantity and excellent quality of fertile mucus. This allowed women to pinpoint the day of ovulation with astonishing precision.

The Smartphone Technology teamed up with FemCap, ultimately providing women with an unprecedentedly accurate prediction of their ovulation day. This new method established a three-day window for conception and eight days for contraception (**Figure 15**).

Women reported that FemCap allowed them to collect large amounts of top-notch cervical secretions that resembled clean egg whites; moreover, these could be stretched up to 2 inches before breaking. This simple, affordable strategy can maximize success rates when trying to conceive or avoid pregnancy among healthy women with regular menstrual cycles.

Synergy created between the FemCap and a Smartphone application (**Figure 14**) provides the safest and most cost-effective birth control without side effects. Investigators and nurses should be encouraged to validate this pilot study.

7. Stress urinary incontinence

Stress Urinary Incontinence (SUI) is prevalent among women of all ages, particularly menopausal women. Women are embarrassed to complain about stress incontinence and silently endure the inconvenience and shame. The (SUI) is under-reported by women, which leads to under-diagnosis and under-treatment [24].

A woman using the FemCap for contraception reported to the first author that she noticed that on the days she wore the FemCap, for contraception, she did *not* suffer from incontinence. Consequently, she decided to wear the FemCap even when she did not need it for contraception [25–27].

This woman's observation led us to investigate a new usage for the FemCap as an SUI pessary (**Figures 16–18**). The current state of the treatment for SUI is pelvic floor muscle (Kegel) exercises and vaginal pessaries. The most popular is the ring pessary; however, various shapes and sizes (**Figures 19–21**) are now available to hopefully achieve better results before recommending surgery. The most recent are Uresta (**Figure 20**) and Introl, and Revive (**Figure 21**).

We began our analysis by comparing the FemCap with the vaginal ring pessary with support (**Figure 16**). The bowl of the FemCap (**Figures 16** and **17**) is designed to secure itself entirely around and below the cervix thereby preventing it prolapse. Additionally, its rim fits closely into the fornices, providing support to the bladder neck (**Figure 21**). The out flaring of the brim distributes pressure evenly against the vaginal wall, the cystocele and over the mid- urethra to restore the anatomy of the cystocele and to straighten the urethra. The FemCap offers a unique advantage when treating or preventing Stress Urinary Incontinence.

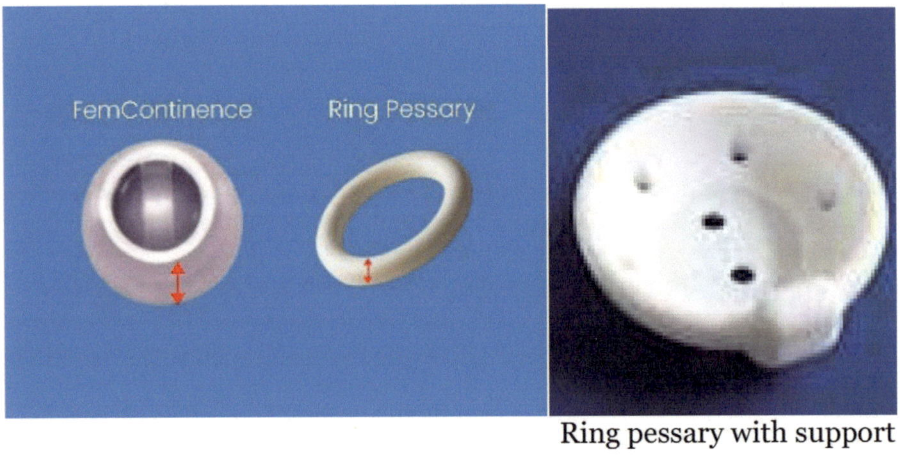

Figure 16.
Ring pessary with support.

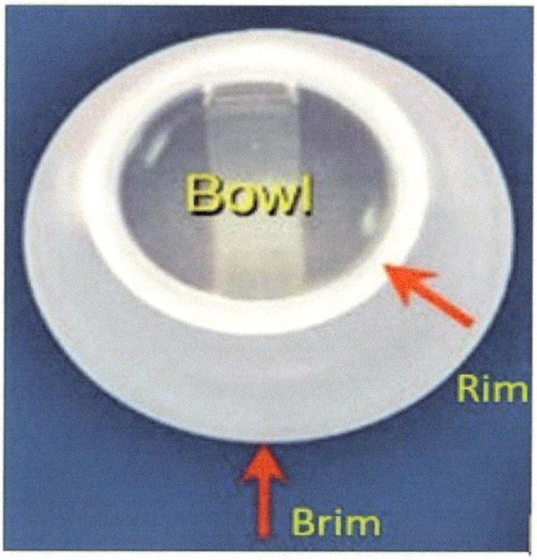

Figure 17.
FemContinence pessary.

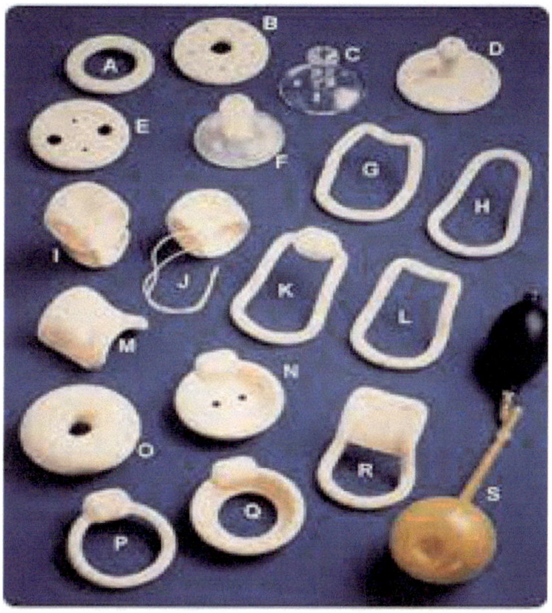

Figure 18.
Vaginal pessaries.

Unlike the ring pessary with support, that usually have a metal knob (**Figure 16**) The FemCap is composed entirely of soft, pliable material. The knob and the rim of the ring pessary with support has an internal metal to exert pressure against the Cystocele and the urethra (**Figures 16** and **20**).

The investigators, Alfred Shihata and Birgit Linderoth, Midwife of Falun of Sweden, did investigate the feasibility of using the FemCap to manage SUI (**Figure 21**) [28].

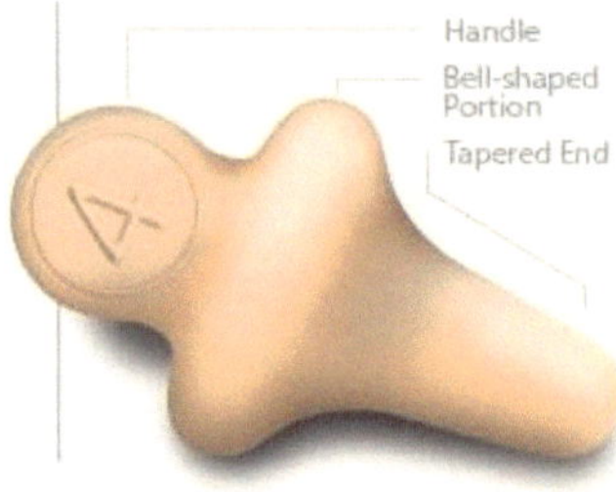

Figure 19.
Courtesy of Uresta.

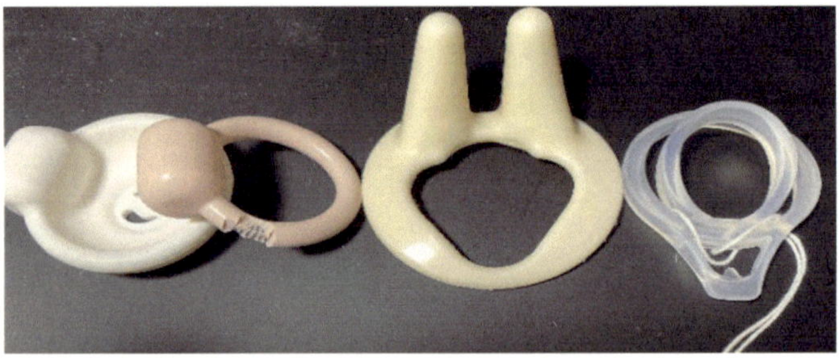

Figure 20.
Ring pessary with support & knob, introl, revive.

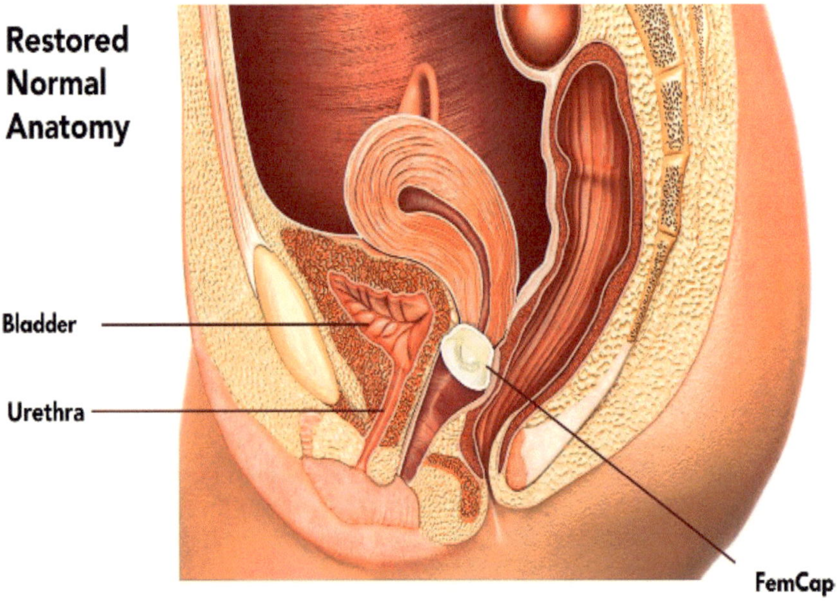

Figure 21.
FemCap Restores Anatomy.

The Current management of mild to moderate SUI is Kegel exercise and ring pessary. We conducted a limited pilot study for 2 weeks to validate the experience of the woman who used the FemCap to control her Stress incontinence. We were pleasantly surprised to validate her experience [29]. We were encouraged and decided to expand the study into Sweden and increase the number of participants [28]. It is worth mentioning that we enrolled 118 women in a very short time.

This study protocol included women with mild to moderate SUI, but those with severe incontinence or 3rd-degree prolapse were excluded.

We asked women to record each episode of incontinence and what precipitated it for one week before using the FemCap, (**Table 2**), as the women's her own control.

We instructed women to follow the same protocol above while using the FemCap (**Table 3**). That Shows the same woman's experience while using FemContinence (FemCap).

7.1 Results

99 women completed the study; 85 were completely dry while using the FemCap. Nine (9) women were partially dry, and 5 women were not satisfied with the results. Ninety-four women, including the partially dry said, they would like to use the FemContinence if available. No side effects were reported by the participants, and pelvic examinations did not show any erosion or ulceration of the vagina. (**Tables 2** and **3**) are an example of a woman who became completely dry [28].

FemCap Stress Urinary						
Incontinence Study by Dr. Alfred Shihata				Questions? Call Us: (858) 922–7673 &$$$;		
Name: Emma from Sweden				Date Before using Femcap:		
How many times per day you have stress incontinence, during the last week BEFORE using the FemCap you when you:						
	Mon	**Tues**	**Wed**	**Thurs**	**Fri**	**Sat**
Cough	2	2	1	3	3	2
Sneeze	3	1	2	2	3	3
Laugh	1	2	1	1	1	1
Stand up	1	3	2	2	2	2
Get out of a car	1	2	3	3	2	3
Lift something heavy	1	2	2	2	1	2
Exercise	3	1	3	2	2	2
Do you wear a pad?	Yes	Yes	Yes	Yes	Yes	Yes
You should insert the FemCap first thing in the morning*. Do not remove it until bedtime and then wash and store it in container until you use it the next morning.						
**If you are using FemCap for birth control use spermicide* *If you are using FemCap for incontinence only use with a water soluble lubricant.*						

Table 2.
Incontinence tracker the week before trying FemContinence.

Date After using FemCap:

How many times per day you have stress incontinence, during the second weeks while using the FemCap:

	Mon	Tues	Wed	Thurs	Fri	Sat	Sun
Cough	0	0	0	0	0	0	0
Sneeze							
Laugh							
Stand up	↓	↓	↓	↓	↓	↓	↓
Get out of a car							
Lift something heavy							
Exercise							
Do you still wear a pad?	Yes	Yes	Yes	No	No	No	No

1. Did have any side effects from the FemCap?
2. Will you consider using the FemCap in the Future to control your (SUI)?
3. Comments I did not have leakage when jumping on the trampoline while using the FemCap, Coughing and sneezing no longer was an issue when I had a cold while using FemCap

Table 3.
Vaginal drug delivery.

7.2 Conclusion

The innovative *FemContinence* (FemCap) device provides a safe, reusable, and self-administered treatment to help manage stress urinary incontinence. The FemCap was able to restore the anatomical structure of the bladder, the bladder neck, and the urethra. Research has revealed that in 85% of cases, this device reduced or eliminated symptoms that negatively impact the overall quality of life. This presents an ideal, low-cost, non-invasive solution for clinicians treating a condition often unspoken about. Further clinical trials should be conducted to verify these results.

Due to the small number of the participants and limitation of this study we welcome any investigator who would like to validate this study. As a token of our appreciation, we will provide all the FemCap (FemContince) free of charge for treating or preventing mild to moderate Stress Urinary Incontinence (SUI). We would not have achieved this result unless the FemCap did restore and maintain the anatomy and by supporting the bladder neck and straighten the urethra and thereby made the urethral sphincters competent.

8. Vaginal drug delivery by the FemCap

Millions of women have used and still using vaginal applicators to introduce creams and gels into the vagina. The regular rhythmic contraction of the vagina is designed to rid itself of menstrual blood and cervical discharges, as well as any treatment-oriented vaginal creams that could be rendered them less effective through these natural forces (**Figures 22** and **23**).

Video 4 (https://www.youtube.com/watch?v=6JNFIOoXeLI) describe the alternative to the currently available vaginal Applicator.

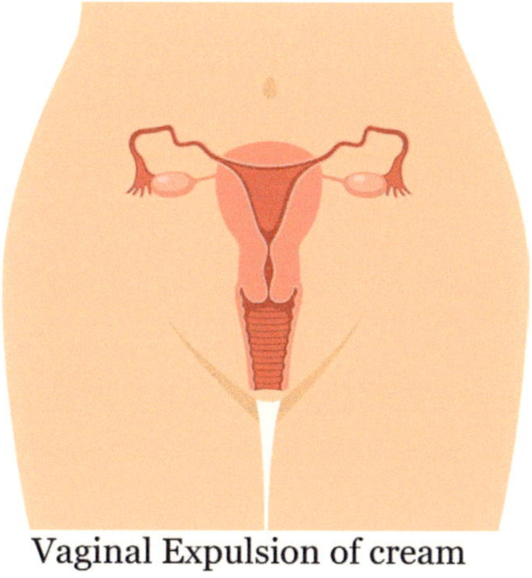

Figure 22.
Vaginal expulsion of cream.

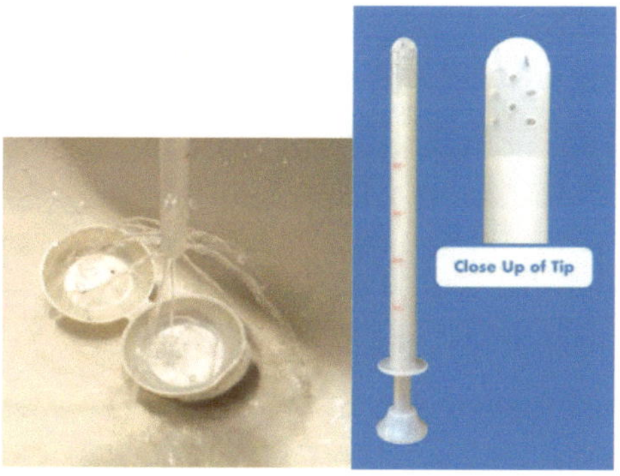

Figure 23.
Shower-head applicator.

The first author developed a showerhead applicator for better distribution and retention of therapeutic vaginal medications. Unfortunately, the vagina did expel the cream rendering them less effective.

The primary focus of this study was to analyze the possibility of offering women an alternative to traditional vaginal applicators and investigate how long FemCap, a new cervical barrier, could keep therapeutic preparations in contact with the cervix and vagina. We wanted to see whether FemCap could effectively treat Bacterial Vaginosis, Candida infections, and some sexually transmitted diseases topically. To prove this concept, we recruited 40 women to insert a stained gel with Gentian violet into the vaginas.

To assess the efficacy of the FemCap device, we randomized women into two groups. Group A of 20 women used a vaginal applicator as the control, and group B employed the FemCap to insert the identical gel into their vaginas. Pads were provided for monitoring any expulsion of the gel while using the traditional applicators and the FemCap. We photographed the cervix and the vagina at 12 and 24 hours.

(See **Figure 24**).

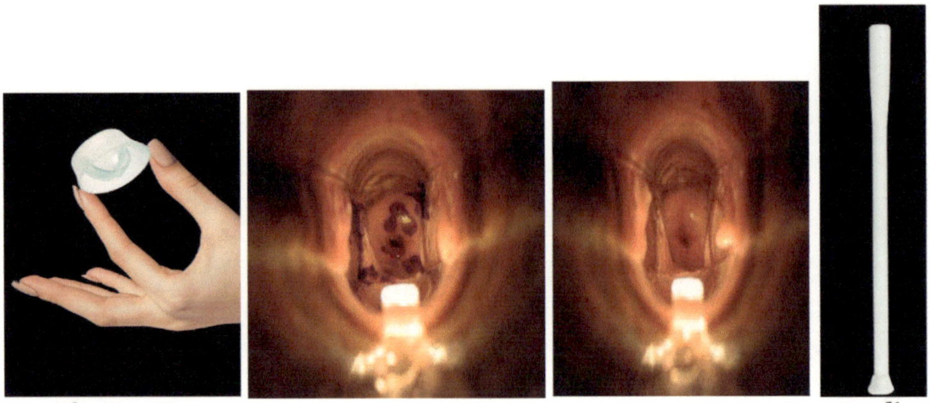

Figure 24.
The FemCap retained stain over 24 hours vs. The applicator.

8.1 Results

During the study, no adverse effects were noted among participants in either group that used the stained gel. Interestingly, several women reported leakage while using a vaginal applicator. While none of the women who used the FemCap had any leakage. Upon examination of cervical photographs taken 12 hours and 24 hours after insertion. Women who used the vaginal applicators had no visible stain after 12 hours. The Stain was visible over the cervix, 24 hours after insertion, with the FemCap.

8.2 Conclusion

This pilot study results showed that, applications of vaginal preparations by the FemCap into the vagina will have better retention and distribution than if it were applied with vaginal applicator.

Further research should investigate whether FemCap can effectively treat ailments such as bacterial vaginosis, candida, and some STIs like gonorrhea and chlamydia topically.

Acknowledgements

This research chapter is written at the request of MS. Tea Jurcic, Author Service Manager of IntechOpen of London. We are indebted to the women who participated in the research study, we thank Dr. Steven Brody, who co-authored and edited this manuscript, and Ms. Birgit Linderoth, a Midwife from Falun, Sweden, who volunteered to enroll her patients in the trials. No funding was requested or received from any institution. We wish to Thank Mr. Sam Awada for donating the FemCap devices. The authors are responsible for the contents of this chapter.

DOI: http://dx.doi.org/10.5772/intechopen.112255

Author details

Alfred A. Shihata[1*], Steven A. Brody[2] and Birgit Linderoth[3]

1 Scripps Institution of Medicine and Science San Diego, Del Mar, CA, USA

2 LifeSpan Medical Institute San Diego, CA, USA

3 Midwife, Falun, Sweden

*Address all correspondence to: alfred@femcap.com

References

[1] Averbach SH, Gravitt PE, Nowak RG, Celentano DD, Dunbar MS, Morrison CS, et al. The association between cervical human papillomavirus infection and HIV acquisition among women in Zimbabwe. AIDS. 2010;**24**(7):1035-1042. DOI: 10.1097/qad.0b013e3283377973

[2] Alfred Shihata, Steven Brody. HIV/STIs and pregnancy prevention, using a cervical barrier and Microbicide.

[3] US patent NO:5,207232 New barrier Contraceptive device FemCap

[4] US patent No 5,778,886 Vaginal compositions combining a spermicidal agent and a peroxygen compound.

[5] https://femcap.com/resources_assets/news-articles/medical_news.htm#WHCJ

[6] Shoupe D, Kjos S. The Handbook of Contraception, Barrier Contraceptives Chapter 10. Humana Press; 2006. pp. 147-177

[7] Carcio H, Clarke SM, Koeniger-Donohue R. Advanced Health Assessment of Women: Clinical Skills and Procedures Chapter 15 the FemCap. Springer. Publishing Company; 2010. pp. 271-278

[8] Scan-Jan-1244-2022.pdf (femcap.com) Advanced Health Assessment of Women.

[9] Shihata AA, Trussell J. New female intravaginal barrier contraceptive device preliminary clinical trial. Contraception. 1991;**44**(1):11-19

[10] Mauck C, Baker J, Barr S, et al. Phase I study of FemCap used with and without spermicide: Postcoital testing. Contraception. 1997;**56**:111-111

[11] Mauck C, Callahan M, Weiner D, et al. A comparative study of the safety and efficacy of FemCap, a new vaginal barrier contraceptive, and the Ortho all-flex® diaphragm. Contraception. 1999;**60**:71-80.6

[12] Shihata A. The FemCap™, a new contraceptive choice. The European Journal of Contraception and Reproductive Health Care. 1998;**3**:160-166

[13] Collins WP. The evolution of reference methods to monitor ovulation prediction. American Journal of Obstetrics and Gynaecology. 1991;**165**:1994-1996

[14] Wolcox A, Weinberg M, Baird D. Timing of sexual intercourse in relation to ovulation. Effects on the Probability of Conception, Survival of the Pregnancy, and Sex of the Baby The New England Journal of Medicine. 1995;**333**:1517-1521

[15] Shihata A, Brody S. Novel approach for women to identify the precise day of ovulation to conceive or contracept. International Journal of Medical Science and Health Research. 2020;**4**(3)

[16] Pyper CMM. Fertility Awareness & Natural Family Planning. The European Journal of Contraception & Reproductive Health Care. 1997;**2**:131-146

[17] Billings JJ. Cervical mucus: The biological marker of fertility and infertility. International Journal of Fertility. 1987;**26**:181

[18] Marshall. The Infertile Period–Principles and Practice. London: Darton, Longman and Todd; 1963

[19] Clubb E, Knight J. Fertility–Fertility Awareness and Natural Family Planning. 3rd ed. David & Charles; 1996

[20] Arevalo M, Sinai I, Jennings V. A fixed formula to define the fertile window of the menstrual cycle as the basis of a simple method of NFP. Contraception. 1999;**60**:357-360

[21] Odeblad E. Cervical mucus and their functions. Journal of the Irish Colleges of Physicians and Surgeons. 1997;**26**(1)

[22] Fordney-Settlage D. A review of cervical mucus and sperm interactions in humans. International Journal of Fertility. 1981;**26**:161-169

[23] Shihata A. New FDA approved woman-controlled, latex-free barrier contraceptive device "FemCap™". Fertil Steril. International Congress Series 1271. 2004;**05**(103):303-330

[24] Viera AJ, Larkins-Pettigrew M. Practical use of the pessary [published correction appears in Am fam physician 2002 Jul 1;66(1):30]. American Family Physician. 2000;**61**(9):2719-2729

[25] Al-Shaikh G, Syed S, Osman S, Bogis A, Al-Badr A. Pessary use in stress urinary incontinence: A review of advantages, complications, patient satisfaction, and quality of life. International Journal of Womens Health. 2018;**10**:195-201. Published 2018 Apr 17. DOI: 10.2147/IJWH.S152616

[26] Jones K, Harmanli O. Pessary use in pelvic organ prolapse and urinary incontinence. Reviews in Obstetrics & Gynecology. 2010. Retrieved from: https://www.ncbi.nlm.nih.gov/pmc/articles/PMC2876320/

[27] Alfred A. Shihata et al. Multipurpose, reusable, female contraceptive device that enhances the effectiveness of fertility awareness methods and controls stress incontinence. Medical Research Archives, [S.l.]. 2020. ISSN 2375-1924

[28] Alfred S. Ongoing research for managing stress urinary incontinence in women with a FDA approved device, the FemCap™, ww.opastonline.com. International Journal of Women's Health Care. 2021;**6**(1):97. https://www.opastpublishers.com/open-access-articles/ongoing-research-for-managing-stress-urinary-incontinence-in-women-with-a-fda-approved-device-the-femcap.pdf

[29] Alfred S. Successful Management of Stress Urinary Incontinence in women by a contraceptive device FemCap™ pilot study, www.opastonline.com. International Journal of Women's Health Care. 2020;**5**(4):81. https://www.opastpublishers.com/open-access-articles/successful-management-of-stress-urinary-incontinence-in-women-by-a-contraceptive-device-femcap-pilot-study.pdf

Chapter 6

Barrier Methods of Contraception

Naana Boadiwaa Asante, Jude Anim and Raida Koray

Abstract

Barrier methods of contraception prevent the exchange of bodily fluids such as semen, vaginal and anal secretions, and blood between partners during intercourse. Thus, the primary function of these methods of contraception is pregnancy prevention. Some, such as internal and external condoms, provide protection against sexually transmitted infections (STIs) as well. Barrier methods of contraception include condoms (external and internal), diaphragm, cervical cap, contraceptive gel, spermicide, and contraceptive sponge. Since they are non-hormonal and have no systemic effects, these are alternatives for women who cannot use hormonal contraceptives due to certain medical conditions or medications prescribed. The efficacy of these methods of contraception is contingent on their correct and consistent use. This chapter aims to discuss the various barrier methods, their usage, mechanisms of action, advantages, and disadvantages as well as the comparison of some of these methods to one another.

Keywords: barrier methods, contraception, non-hormonal, sexually transmitted infection, efficacy

1. Introduction

Contraception has been around for some centuries now. Using various techniques to prevent pregnancy, ancient writings dating back to 1850 BC recorded the insertion of various substances into the vagina. Substances such as crocodile dung, gum, honey, and acacia were used. At that time, it was believed that these substances created a hostile environment for sperm to survive [1]. Another well-known method dating back to centuries which is still being used is coitus interruptus (withdrawal method). The effectiveness of withdrawal is dependent on timing, self-control, and apt removal of the penis before ejaculating. Due to the high failure rates of this method, other methods had to be devised to address contraception [2]. As medicine extended its tentacles to address contraception, the main points of focus were efficiency, efficacy, mechanism of action, and the failure rates of each device and pill created.

Contraception can be classified into barrier and non-barrier methods. Barrier methods act as blockages that prevent sperms from reaching the egg [1]. Barrier methods of contraception which are the focus of this chapter have been recognized many centuries ago. As early as the 18th and 19th centuries, items such as leaves, sponges, and lemons were used to block sperm from entering the uterus [3]. For instance, some ancient Egyptian arts display men with decorative coverings of their penises [3]. Just like the withdrawal method which has a high failure rate, these barrier methods were to some extent unreliable because of their fragility, nature, and low to no proficiency rate. Over time, barrier methods including spermicides, condoms, diaphragms, cervical caps, and contraceptive gels and sponges were discovered. The game changer for barrier methods to be unleashed was when rubber was discovered in 1839 by Hancock and Goodyear [3]. With this discovery, many of the barrier methods from the 19th century up until now were made of rubber which made them inexpensive and easily accessible to many. On a wide scale, even though barrier methods can interrupt pregnancy, most are not effective in protecting against sexually transmitted diseases.

The vast types of barrier methods give an individual many options to birth control depending on the conduciveness of lifestyle, accessibility, risk, consistency, and usage. Other factors to consider in selecting a barrier method include allergies, bouts of sexual encounters, duration, and frequency of the device's usage. Some barrier methods require a physician's discretion while others can be purchased over the counter. Even in some cases, the efficiency of contraception can be achieved by the combination of various barrier methods. Advantageously over non-barrier methods, barrier methods can be used intermittently and possibly overcome systemic side effects [1]. In this book chapter, we will discuss the various barrier methods, their mechanism of action, efficacy, advantages, and disadvantages.

2. External (male) condoms

2.1 Introduction

It is a thin protective sheath worn over an erect penis during intercourse [4]. External condoms reduce the likelihood of unintended pregnancy and transmission of sexually transmitted infections (STIs) when used correctly and during every sexual activity [4].

2.2 Types of external condoms

External condoms are made from various materials and come in different shapes, sizes, thicknesses, colors, flavors, and with or without reservoir tips that collect semen. They may or may not contain lubricants or spermicides [5, 6].

2.2.1 Latex condoms

Most condoms manufactured commercially are made of latex. They are less expensive and have higher tensile strength than non-latex condoms. Latex condoms are more effective than non-latex condoms at protecting against all common types of STIs with correct and consistent use [7]. Although the advantages of latex have made it the most preferred material for condoms, it has a few drawbacks. Latex condoms can trigger an allergic reaction in people who are allergic to latex [1, 4, 8] and are degraded by oil-based lubricants; therefore, they should not be used in conjunction with oil-based lubricants [1, 4, 9].

2.2.2 Non-latex condoms

Non-latex condoms can be made from lambskin and synthetic materials such as polyurethane, silicone, or polyisoprene [1, 4]. Non-latex condoms are an alternative for individuals who are allergic to latex [1, 4, 8]. Polyurethane condoms do not stretch like latex or polyisoprene, making them more susceptible to slippage and breakage. Polyurethane condoms are thinner and conduct heat better than latex and polyisoprene which may enhance sensitivity. Polyurethane condoms can be used with both water-based and oil-based lubricants. In contrast to polyurethane condoms, polyisoprene condoms are cheaper, stretchier, thicker, conduct heat poorly, and are incompatible with oil-based lubricants [1]. Lambskin condoms are manufactured from the intestine of a lamb and are not as common as the other external condoms [1, 4, 8], and can be used with any type of lubricant [6]. Because of their porous nature, viruses such as HIV, hepatitis, and herpes simplex as well as bacteria such as gonorrhea can easily pass through; thus, they do not offer protection against STIs. They are only effective for preventing pregnancy [1, 4, 8].

2.3 Mechanism of action

It functions by creating a physical barrier that prevents the entry of semen into the vagina. Also, it prevents direct contact with genital lesions, secretions from the penis, vagina, anus, and subclinical viral shedding on the genitals. Thus, pregnancy as well as STIs like HIV can be prevented [4, 5].

2.4 How to put on and remove an external condom

- For every sexual encounter, a new condom should be used [4, 7].
- Always use the right condom size.
- Before you open the package, inspect it, and check the expiration date. Do not use it if it is expired, torn, or damaged.
- Carefully open one end of the condom package. Avoid using your teeth or objects that can tear the condom.
- With the rolled side of the condom out, place the condom on the tip of the erect penis and leave about ½ inch space at the top to collect semen.
- Pinch the tip of the condom with one hand to get rid of trapped air.
- With the other hand, unroll the condom to fully cover the shaft of the erect penis.
- After ejaculation, make sure you withdraw the penis from the other partner's body while it is still erect to prevent spillage of semen. Hold the rim of the condom when withdrawing the penis.
- Remove the condom, wrap it in tissue or plastic bag and dispose of it in a bin.

2.5 Efficacy

The most important factor in determining the efficacy of condom use is correct and consistent use [4, 8]. External condoms are highly efficacious in pregnancy prevention, with just about 2% of women becoming pregnant within the first year of perfect use of condoms and approximately 13% being pregnant within the first year of typical use [4, 10]. Perfect use of condoms refers to correct and consistent usage while typical use refers to the way most people use them [11]. With correct and consistent usage, external condoms are estimated to be 80–95% effective in preventing the spread of HIV and other STIs [4].

2.6 Advantages

- External condoms are safe to use with no systemic side effects.
- They provide effective protection against STIs, including HIV by acting as a physical barrier that prevents the exchange of bodily fluids [4].
- They are easy to use and do not require special training or skills.
- They are widely available to individuals without a prescription. They can be obtained from pharmacies, clinics, supermarkets, convenience stores and gas stations [6, 12].
- They are relatively inexpensive, and even freely distributed at condom distribution programmes [6].
- They are reversible methods of contraception that do not interfere with fertility for both partners [4].
- For some men, wearing thicker condoms can help prevent premature ejaculation by reducing sensitivity in the penis and improving penile erection [13].

2.7 Disadvantages

- The use of regular condoms is a challenge for individuals who are allergic to latex. Non-latex condoms are relatively expensive and not as effective as latex condoms.
- Concerns about reduced sensitivity during sexual intercourse are frequently expressed by couples who use condoms [6, 12].
- Some users have difficulty maintaining an erection while wearing condoms [6].
- It can be difficult to withdraw the penis from the vagina before it becomes flaccid after ejaculation, which can cause condom slippage and semen discharge into the vagina [12].
- Condoms can tear or break during intercourse and may result in an unwanted pregnancy or exposure to STIs. Some of the factors associated with condom breakage are excessive friction during sex, longer duration of intercourse, incorrect usage, using the wrong size, use of oil-based lubricants, and reuse of condoms [9, 13, 14]. Oil-based lubricants can impair the integrity of latex condoms [9].

3. Internal (female) condoms

3.1 Introduction

Internal condoms are the only female-controlled contraceptive method that has been proven to reduce the likelihood of both unintended pregnancy as well as transmission of sexually transmitted infections (STIs). It is a tool for empowering women as it bolsters their sexual confidence and offers them more control over their reproductive health.

Typically, an internal condom consists of a soft sheath and two flexible rings. The closed end of the sheath has an inner ring which is inserted vaginally. An outer ring at the open end lies outside the vagina after insertion [15]. It is intended for only one-time use. In contrast to external condoms, internal condoms can be inserted at any time up to 8 hours prior to intercourse [4]. Note: Internal and external condoms should not be used concurrently, as friction between the two can result in slippage or tearing [4].

3.2 Types of internal condoms

3.2.1 Polyurethane condoms (FC1)

FC1, which is no longer commercially available, was made of Polyurethane. They were the first generation of internal condoms that was approved by the United States Food and Drug Administration (USFDA) in 1993 [15]. However, polyurethane condoms have been replaced by newer versions of female condoms that are less expensive and have high acceptance rates. Although internal condoms available on the market today differ in designs and materials, they have many functional and structural similarities [15]. It was approximately 17 cm long and pre-lubricated with dimethicone, a silicone-based lubricant [15].

3.2.2 FC2

The Femidom female condom (FC2), which replaced the FC1, is just as efficacious as its predecessor but is made of nitrile and does not have a seam. It makes less noise than FC1 during intercourse [15]. It is pre-lubricated with a silicone-based lubricant on both the interior and exterior. It is the only commercially available internal condom approved by the FDA. It has received CE marking and approval by the WHO [16]. Studies comparing FC2 and FC1 found that the FC2 was on par with the FC1 in terms of patient's acceptability, breakage, slippage, and invagination but sold at a lower price [15, 17].

3.2.3 VA w.o.w (worn of women)

L'amour, Condom Feminine, and Reddy FC are some of the brand names under which it is sold. It is made of latex, just like external condoms. Its unique design features a medical-grade sponge anchored to its closed end for insertion and a triangular frame at the open end which lies outside the vagina. It has received CE Marking and is currently being evaluated by the WHO [16, 17].

3.2.4 The Woman's condom

The PATH (Program for Appropriate Technology in Health) Women's condom is manufactured with polyurethane and has an insertion capsule that dissolves inside the vagina. It is not pre-lubricated; rather, a water-based lubricant is included in the package that the user must apply. The presence of hydrophilic areas on the condom allows it to adhere lightly to the walls of the vagina, which keeps the condom in place [16, 17]. Data from a single-arm study carried out in China to evaluate the performance of WC in terms of function and safety, were consistent with data already available on the effectiveness of the other internal condoms, indicating that the WC performs as well as the other internal condoms [18]. It has CE marking and is currently under review by the WHO [16].

3.2.5 Phoenurse (PFC)

It is a polyurethane condom that comes pre-lubricated with a water or silicone-based lubricant and has an insertion tool attached to the inner ring [15, 19]. It is only distributed in China, [15, 19, 20] and received approval from the China State Food and Drug Administration (CFDA) only [15, 19]. In a randomized control trial conducted in China, FC2 was preferred over PFC in terms of lubrication, color, and overall fit [21]. Another study conducted in China revealed that breakage, misdirection of the penis, and slippage were significantly more common with the PFC than with the FC2 [22]. It has received only CE marking [16].

3.2.6 Natural latex female condom (cupid FC and cupid FC2)

It is made of natural latex and pre-lubricated with a silicone-based lubricant. It also has a medical-grade polyurethane sponge attached to the inner ring for insertion and stability and has an octagonal outer ring. The only differences between Cupid2 and Cupid® are that Cupid2 is a bit shorter and has a smaller sponge [19]. In a randomized noninferiority clinical trial, Cupid2 and FC2 had similar clinical failure rates in terms of invagination, clinical breakage, penile misdirection, and slippage [23]. It has received CE marking and approval by the WHO [16].

3.2.7 Panty female condoms

It is composed of a reusable nylon woman's panty and a condom sheath. The panty serves as the outer ring and secures the condom sheath during intercourse. The condom sheath must be replaced following each use. A pilot study conducted in South Africa revealed that, the clinical failure rate of the Panty Condom in terms of clinical breakage, misdirection, slippage, and invagination was about twice that seen in functionality studies of the other internal condoms [24].

3.3 Mechanism of action

Internal condoms are sheaths that line the vagina acting as physical barriers that prevent the introduction of sperms directly into the female reproductive tract, thereby preventing pregnancy. Also, they prevent the transmission of sexually transmitted infections by preventing the exchange of genital secretions [4].

3.4 How to put on an internal condom

1. For every sexual intercourse, a new condom should be used.

2. Inspect the package and check the expiration date. If it is expired, torn, or damaged, do not use it.

3. Wash your hands and carefully open one end of the condom. Avoid using your teeth, fingernails, or objects that can damage the condom.

4. When inserting the condom, you can squat, lie down, or sit.

5. Squeeze the inner ring of the condom with your thumb and index finger and insert it into the vagina. Push it deep with one finger until it rests against the cervix while ensuring that the condom is not twisted. The outer ring should lie outside the vagina.

6. Direct the penis into the opening of the condom. If the penis slips between the condom and the vaginal wall, you must withdraw and try again, or if the outer ring is pushed into the vagina, re-adjust the ring, and try again.

7. After intercourse, hold the outer ring and gently twist it to prevent the semen from spilling out, and then gently pull the condom out of the vagina.

8. Wrap the used condom in tissue or plastic bag and throw it into a bin. Do not reuse [4].

3.5 Efficacy

During the first year of using internal condoms, approximately 5% of women will get pregnant with perfect use and about 21% of women will get pregnant with typical use [4]. These estimated failure rates are from studies conducted on the efficacy of FC1. Currently, there is no specific data on FC2 condoms' ability to prevent pregnancy and STIs. Since the FC2 condom shares many characteristics with the FC1 condom, including its functionality and design, its effectiveness in preventing pregnancy and STIs is assumed to be comparable to that of the FC1 [15, 19]. Although in vitro studies have suggested that internal condoms are impermeable to HIV and other STIs, there are limited clinical studies that have evaluated the internal condom's ability to prevent HIV transmission.

3.6 Advantages

- Internal condoms are non-hormonal therefore they do not have systemic side effects or interfere with medications. As a result, they are an alternative for individuals with contraindications to hormonal contraceptives.

- Some internal condoms are latex-free and can be used by individuals with latex allergy.

- It is a simple and reversible method of contraception that does not cause a delay in the return of fertility when the method is discontinued.

- It is safe to use while breastfeeding.

- Internal condoms are available over the counter.

- It can be worn up to 8 hours before sex therefore there's no need to rush which can kill the mood.

- The external ring may stimulate the clitoris in some women during intercourse, thus enhancing sexual arousal.
- It provides effective protection against pregnancy and STIs as it offers broader coverage of the external genitalia [4, 12].

3.7 Disadvantages

- Internal condoms can be a bit difficult to insert and remove for some women.
- Feeling of discomfort during insertion
- It may slip into the vagina during intercourse and interfere with the spontaneity of sexual experience.
- It can make unpleasant noise during intercourse.
- It is generally more expensive and not widely available as external condoms.
- It has a higher failure rate in preventing pregnancy compared with most other female contraceptive methods and the external condom.
- Internal condoms are not as widely available as external condoms.
- Internal condoms have lower acceptance rates due to factors such as feeling of discomfort during insertion, rejection by the opposite sex, misconception of effectiveness and high cost.

3.8 Internal condoms vs. external condoms

- Internal condoms can be worn for up to 8 hours prior to intercourse while external condoms are only worn just before initiating intercourse.
- One does not require an erection to put on an internal condom; it can be inserted vaginally or anally while external condoms can only be worn over an erected penis.
- Internal condoms are not as widely available as external condoms.
- Internal condoms have higher failure rates compared to external condoms.

4. Diaphragms

4.1 Introduction

Diaphragms are shallow silicone dome-shaped cups with a flexible rim that are inserted into the vagina to cover the cervix. Diaphragms are reusable for up to two years and are available in various sizes– single-size and multisize. The single-size diaphragm, also known as the Caya diaphragm, is the standard and measures about 75 mm long by 67 mm wide. It does not require traditional fitting by a healthcare provider [4, 25]. Instructions are easily applicable by the user. Multisided diaphragms are diaphragm-fitting kit that is used by the clinician to figure out which best fits the woman's anatomy and to educate patients on how to insert and remove the device without complications [4, 25]. Notably, diaphragms are often used with contraceptive gels to increase its efficacy. Usually used with a spermicide, it provides both a chemical and physical barrier to the sperm. Males condoms can be used at the same time a woman uses a diaphragm to increase contraceptive effectiveness and accuracy.

4.2 Mechanism of action

The diaphragm works by covering the cervix, therefore, preventing sperms from getting through the cervix to the uterus. With the combination of the contraceptive gel or spermicide, the sperms are held back by the shallow silicone-shaped dome in the cervix, and the sperms are killed by the spermicide. The diaphragm consists of little bumps on the outer layer which help grip the device around the cervix and for easier insertion into the vagina with a grip or a squeeze [4, 25].

4.3 How it is used

A woman can learn to use a diaphragm herself. It is simple to insert without any complications.

- First, the user washes her hands thoroughly with soap and water.
- Checks the diaphragm for any damages such as holes, tears or cracks each time she uses the device.
- Check the expiration date of the spermicide, water lubricant, or contraceptive gel to avoid using an expired product.
- The user pinches the diaphragm together with both her thumb and index finger; then places a line of contraceptive gel in each fold and slightly on the front rim to enable easy insertion into the vagina without friction.
- The user chooses a comfortable position such as lying down, standing with one leg up, or squatting.
- The device is inserted with the front rim first in the direction of the tailbone by pushing it all the way in as her finger can reach. Then she pushes the front edge up to tuck it behind her pubic bone. If she does not aim the diaphragm toward her tailbone, it will not be in the right place.
- To be sure the diaphragm is correctly fixed, she can feel her cervix with her finger to be sure that the cervix is completely covered by the diaphragm.
- If the position of the diaphragm feels uncomfortable, she can take it out and reinsert it.

- Note, the diaphragm should remain in the vagina for at least 6 hours after having coitus but not more than 24 hours [4].
- For multiple coital acts, the diaphragm should be in the right position and additional spermicide should be inserted in front of the diaphragm before having sex.
- Leaving the diaphragm in place for more than 24 hours can cause bad odor, unusual vaginal discharge, urinary tract infections, and toxic shock syndrome.
- If the diaphragm is too large, the user may not be able to insert it completely which may feel uncomfortable. If it is too small, it may not completely cover up the cervix.
- Women who just had a baby will have to wait for 6 weeks before they can use this device [4, 26].

4.3.1 To remove the diaphragm

- Wash your hands thoroughly with soap and water.
- Insert a finger into the vagina until the rim of the diaphragm is felt.
- Calmly slide a finger under the rim and pull the diaphragm down and out.
- Wash the diaphragm with soap and water, air dry the device in its open case at room temperature and store it for later use. This device can be used for up to 2 years [4].

4.4 Efficacy

With consistent and correct use together with spermicide, the failure rate for typical use is 12% and that for perfect use is 6%. In comparison to other contraceptive methods such as cervical cap and contraceptive sponge, the diaphragm is more effective and can be used for a longer time (up to 2 years) [25, 27].

4.5 Advantages

- Diaphragms can be inserted ahead of time. In due process, the woman can prepare well before any sexual encounter with less stress and surprises. Also, with the ample time to utilize the device (inserted at least 6 hours but removed before 24 hours), the partners can use the device with multiple bouts of sexual encounters in the day.
- It can be reused for up to 2 years.
- After the initial purchase of the diaphragm and its accessories, the only expense left is replacing the spermicide.
- After education and fitting instruction are conveyed by a health professional, there is no need for periodic visits to the clinic for evaluation up until 2 years. It saves time and money.

- Diaphragms do not cause systemic adverse effects. Unlike other contraceptives such as oral contraceptives and implants, diaphragms do not affect the hormonal balance of the user [4, 25, 28].

4.6 Disadvantages

- Just like some contraceptives that need a prescription and education from a licensed health provider, diaphragms are no different. Individuals without access to a clinic or a health professional cannot get this device [4, 25].
- Considered to have a lower efficacy rate compared to other contraceptives such as intrauterine devices such as progestin which have an efficacy rate of 99% [29].
- There are also side effects and complications such as urinary tract infections (UTI), vaginal irritations, and toxic shock.

  syndrome (TSS).

5. Cervical cap

5.1 Introduction

The cervical cap is a reusable silicone cup shaped like a sailor's hat. It is inserted into the vagina before coitus with the dome-shaped area of the cap covering the cervix. Usually, a cervical cap is used with a spermicide to boost its efficacy [4, 28]. The spermicide increases contraception by killing the sperms that come into contact with the cervical cap and reduces the fetid discharge brought on by the continuous use of the cervical cap [4].

5.2 Mechanism of action

The cervical cap fits snugly over the cervix, preventing sperm from entering the uterus. Similar to the mechanism of the diaphragm, the cervical cap blocks the sperm from entering the cervix and the spermicide in the dome kills the sperms. It provides both physical and chemical barriers at the entrance of the cervix.

5.3 To insert a cervical cap

- Wash your hands thoroughly with soap and water.
- Apply one-third of the cap with spermicidal cream to the dome of the cap up to the brim.
- Apply an additional 1/2 teaspoon of spermicide in the groove between the outside of the dome and the brim.
- Choose a comfortable position for insertion. You can decide to lie down, stand with one foot on a chair or squat.
- Locate the cervix using your index and middle finger by placing both in the vagina.

- Firmly press the cervical cap with the dome pointing away from the vagina.
- With one or two fingers, slide the longer part of the brim into the vagina making sure the cervix is completely covered by the cap.
- Leave the cap for up to 48 hours [30].

5.3.1 Remove cervical cap

- Wash your hands thoroughly with soap and water.
- Wait up to 6 hours after sex before removing the cap.
- Squat and slide a finger into the vagina to locate the strap that covers the dome [25].
- Use the tip of your finger to slowly push the dome to break the suction [25].
- Gently pull down on the strap to remove the cap from the vagina.
- With soap and water, wash the cap with soap, and water and let it air dry.

5.4 Efficacy

Women who are nulliparous or who have never given birth vaginally respond best to the cervical cap as a method of contraception. Out of 100 women who will become pregnant with typical use of the cervical cap, only about 13% are nulliparous and about 32% are multiparous. Since the sizes of the cervix alter because of pregnancy and abortion, the small size (22 mm) is usually for patients who have not been pregnant before, while the medium size (26 mm) is for patients who have had an abortion or cesarean delivery and large size (30 mm) for users who have had full term delivery vaginally [25].

5.5 Advantages

- It can be inserted 6 hours before having intercourse, so the woman can prepare adequately.
- It is easily reversible when insertion is uncomfortable.
- It is affordable and can be used for up to 2 years [25, 29].

5.6 Disadvantages

- It is required with every act of intercourse.
- Provides no protection against STIs.
- Has difficult learning insertion and removal instructions.
- Cervical cap cannot be used [31]:

- 8–10 weeks after giving birth.
- 6 weeks after miscarriage or abortion because at that point the cervix is enlarged so it is easier to become pregnant.
- During a menstrual period because it can block normal drainage of blood from the uterus.

5.7 Differences associated with diaphragm and cervix

Cervical caps are smaller than diaphragms, so therefore they fit snugly on the cervix.

Cervical caps can be used for up to 48 hours while diaphragms can be used for 24 hours.

Cervical caps are more expensive than diaphragms.

6. pH regulator contraceptive gel

6.1 Introduction

The contraceptive gel is a formulation that contains lactic acid (18 mg/g), citric acid (10 mg/g), and potassium bitartrate (4 mg/g) as active ingredients. It is marketed under the brand name Phexxi (previously on the market as Amphora and ACIDFORM). It comes in 12 pre-filled applicators, each containing 5 grams of gel, and is available by prescription only. It provides on-demand contraception when used prior to intercourse. It was approved for contraceptive use in 2020. It works better when used in conjunction with other barrier methods like condoms, diaphragms, and cervical caps [29–34].

6.2 Mechanism of action

It works by lowering the pH of the vagina to between 3.5 and 4.5 even in the presence of alkaline semen, creating a more acidic environment that affects the viability and motility of sperms thus preventing fertilization [35].

6.3 How it is used

- Inspect the package and check the expiration date. Do not use it if it is expired or the seal is broken.
- Ensure that you read and follow the instructions on the package carefully.
- Wash your hands thoroughly before opening the pouch.
- Apply one dose into the vagina with the applicator no more than 1 hour prior to intercourse.
- Reapply one dose of gel before each coital act. If there's more than one coital act within an hour, it is recommended to administer a second dose for increased efficacy. Reapplication is necessary if intercourse does not occur within an hour.

- Dispose of the used pre-filled applicator [34, 36]
- Note: It is not effective when used after intercourse.

6.4 Efficacy

The estimated failure rates are 7% within the first year of perfect use and 14% within the first year of typical use. It does not provide users with protection against sexually transmitted infections [7, 35, 37].

6.5 Advantages

- It is non-hormonal.
- It can be applied up to one hour before sex, therefore, it does not interrupt foreplay.
- It can be applied during the menstrual cycle.

6.6 Disadvantages and side effects

- It does not offer protection against STIs.
- Common side effects such as vulvovaginal burning, vulvovaginal itching, vulvovaginal pain, bacterial vaginosis, urinary tract infections, and vaginal yeast infections (candidiasis) were experienced by about 2% of participants in phase 3 of a clinical trial conducted in the United States and were reported to be mild or moderate [36]. Major side effects such as pyelonephritis, cystitis or other upper urinary tract infections were experienced by 0.36% of the participants in phases 1 and 2 of the clinical trial [34].
- In a clinical trial, spouses of participants reported penile irritation [3, 36]

6.7 Contraindications

- It should not be used by women who have a history of recurrent urinary tract infections or urinary tract anomalies [34, 37].
- It is not recommended during pregnancy. According to the FDA, the risk for miscarriage is 15–20% and major birth defects is 2–4% [34].

7. Spermicides

7.1 Introduction

Spermicidal contraceptives contain a spermicidal agent and a carrier. The active ingredient commonly used is nonoxynol-9 which is a surfactant. Currently, nonoxynol-9 and octoxynol-9 are the only FDA-approved spermicidal agents. Spermicidal contraceptives come in a variety of formulations such as gels, creams, jellies, foaming tablets, suppositories, films, and sponges. They can be used alone or combined with condoms, diaphragms, and cervical caps for increased efficacy. They are only effective when utilized prior to intercourse, and are available over the counter [4, 25].

7.2 Mechanism of action

Nonoxynol-9 in spermicidal products damages the cell wall of sperms, impeding their transit from the vagina to the uterus [25].

7.3 How they are used

- Inspect the package and check the expiration date. Do not use it if the package is broken or expired.
- Ensure you have read and understood the instructions on the package.
- Hands must be washed thoroughly with soap under running water.
- Vaginal spermicidal gel and creams can be inserted up to one hour before intercourse.
- It is necessary to insert suppositories, films, and tablets at least 10 minutes before sexual activity to give them enough time to dissolve.
- When using spermicidal foams, you do not have to wait for 10 minutes before having intercourse.
- Reapply the spermicide before each act of intercourse.
- Douching must be avoided since it will affect the efficacy of spermicides and increases the user's risk of contracting STIs.
- Wait for at least six hours after having sex if you want to douche [4, 25].

7.4 Efficacy

Spermicide is one of the least effective means of contraception. For spermicides such as foam, gel, cream, film, suppository, tablets, and jelly, the estimated failure rates with typical use and perfect use are 21% and 16% respectively. Spermicides are ineffective in preventing the transmission of sexually transmitted infections [4].

7.5 Advantages

- They are non-hormonal.
- They are available over the counter.
- They can be easily applied by the user.
- They can be used ahead of time and so do not interfere with foreplay.

- They provide extra lubrication.
- Their use is controlled by women [4, 25].

7.6 Disadvantages

- They do not protect against STIs.
- They have high failure rates therefore must be combined with other barrier methods.
- Side effects such as vaginal and penile irritation.
- Frequent use can cause vaginal lesions which may increase one's risk of HIV infection [4].

7.7 Contraindications

- Women who are allergic to nonoxynol-9.
- HIV-positive women
- Women at high risk of exposure to sexually transmitted infections (STIs) [4, 25].

How does pH contraceptive gel differ from spermicide?

pH contraceptive gel does not contain nonoxynol-9 (N-9) which is the active ingredient in spermicide. N-9 can cause disruption of the epithelial cells of the vagina when used repeatedly which may enhance HIV transmission in high-risk individuals [33, 34].

8. Contraceptive sponge

8.1 Introduction

It is a polyurethane sponge that contains a nonoxynol-9 spermicidal agent and is marketed under the brand name Today sponge. It is available over the counter and does not require to be fitted by a health professional [38].

8.2 Mechanism of action

In addition to the effect nonoxynol-9 has on sperms, the sponge blocks the opening of the cervix and absorbs semen thus preventing the entry of sperms into the uterus [38].

8.3 How it is used

- Inspect the package and check the expiration date. Do not use it if the package is broken or expired.

- Hands must be washed thoroughly with soap under running water.
- Remove the sponge from the package.
- Wet the sponge with clean water and gently squeeze it until it is sudsy. The spermicide becomes only activated when moistened.
- Choose a comfortable position for insertion (squat, lie down, or sit)
- With the dimpled side facing upwards, fold the sides of the sponge inward toward the dimple and insert it and push it as far back into the vagina.
- Ensure the sponge is well positioned by feeling around the outline of the sponge with a finger.
- The sponge can be left in the vagina for up to 24 hours, providing protection throughout that time frame regardless of the number of times the user has.
- The sponge should be left in the vagina for 6 hours after the last coital act before removing.
- The sponge must not be kept in the vagina for longer than 30 hours [38].

8.4 Efficacy

For nulliparous women and multiparous women, the typical use failure rates are 12% and 24%, respectively. It does not offer the user protection against sexually transmitted infections [25, 27].

8.5 Advantages

- It provides 24-hour protection without having the need to replace it following multiple bouts of coitus.
- It is available over the counter and does not require fitting by a health professional.
- It allows spontaneity.
- It is safe and easy to use.
- They provide extra lubrication [38].

8.6 Disadvantages

- Side effects such as vaginal irritation and dryness are commonly experienced.
- The incidence of nonmenstrual toxic shock syndrome has been reported although it is rare [38].

8.7 Contraindications

- Women who have had toxic shock syndrome in the past.
- Those who are allergic to sulphites since the product contains metabisulphite.
- If you or your partner has HIV/AIDS
- Women with a history of an allergic reaction to polyurethane, nonoxynol 9, or this product.
- It cannot be used during the menstrual cycle [38].

9. Conclusion

Barrier methods of contraception are the most effective coitus-dependent contraceptive method for preventing unintended pregnancies and STIs. There are a variety of options with varying levels of efficacy from which one can choose from based on one's preferences and lifestyle. Consistent and correct use are crucial to maximizing their effectiveness irrespective of the method chosen. In contrast to hormonal contraceptives, barrier methods do not cause systemic side effects, therefore they are especially suitable for women with medical conditions that preclude the use of hormonal contraception.

Conflict of interest

None.

Author details

Naana Boadiwaa Asante[1*], Jude Anim[2] and Raida Koray[3]

1 37 Military Hospital, Accra, Ghana

2 Georgia Gwinnett College, Georgia, United States

3 Eastern Regional Hospital, Accra, Ghana

*Address all correspondence to: naanababywaa@hotmail.com;
naanababywaa@gmail.com

References

[1] Colquitt CW, Martin TS. Contraceptive methods: A review of nonbarrier and barrier products. Journal of Pharmacy Practice. 2017;**30**(1):130-135

[2] Withdrawal Method (Coitus Interruptus) - Mayo Clinic [Internet]. [cited 2023 Apr 30]. Available from: https://www.mayoclinic.org/tests-procedures/withdrawal-method/about/pac-20395283#:~:text=Even%20then%2C%20the%20withdrawal%20method,protection%20from%20sexually%20transmitted%20infections

[3] A brief history of contraception [Internet]. Wellcome Collection. 2020. [cited 2023 Apr 30]. Available from: https://wellcomecollection.org/articles/XzqUmxEAACEA5N3w

[4] WHO-JHU-FPHandbook-2022Ed-v221114b.pdf [Internet]. [cited 2023 Apr 2]. Available from: https://fphandbook.org/sites/default/files/WHO-JHU-FPHandbook-2022Ed-v221114b.pdf

[5] Male Condoms. In: Contraceptive Technology [Internet]. [cited 2023 Apr 30]. Available from: http://eknygos.lsmuni.lt/springer/540/232-247.pdf

[6] External (formerly male) Condoms - UpToDate [Internet]. [cited 2023 Apr 2]. Available from: https://www.uptodate.com/contents/external-formerly-male-condoms?csi=44df868c-ebc5-448b-80cf-7d8cd1213830&source=contentShare

[7] Barrier Contraceptives - Women's Health Issues [Internet]. MSD Manual Consumer Version. [cited 2023 Apr 2]. Available from: https://www.msdmanuals.com/home/women-s-health-issues/family-planning/barrier-contraceptives

[8] Gilliam ML, Derman RJ. Barrier methods of contraception. Obstetrics and Gynecology Clinics of North America. 2000;**27**(4):841-858

[9] Steiner M, Piedrahita C, Glover L, Joanis C, Spruyt A, Foldesy R. The impact of lubricants on latex condoms during vaginal intercourse. International Journal of STD & AIDS. 1994;**5**(1):29-36

[10] Contraceptive efficacy: understanding how user and method characteristics play their part | Contraceptive Technology [Internet]. [cited 2023 Mar 14]. Available from: https://contraceptivetechnology.org/contraceptive-efficacy-understanding-how-user-and-method-characteristics-play-their-part/

[11] Majra J. Use of condoms: Clarifying the message. Indian Journal of Community Medicine Official Publications Indian Association Prevents Society Medicine. 2010;**35**(2):362

[12] Condoms - Advantages and Disadvantages [Internet]. [cited 2023 Apr 2]. Available from: https://www.news-medical.net/health/Condoms-Advantages-and-Disadvantages.aspx

[13] Wang Z, Yu J. Efficacy evaluation of thickened condom in the treatment of premature ejaculation. Translational Andrology and Urology. 2022;**11**(2):253-259

[14] Richters J, Gerofi J, Donovan B. Why do condoms break or slip off in use? An exploratory study. International Journal of STD & AIDS. 1995;**6**(1):11-18

[15] Beksinska M, Smit J, Joanis C, Usher-Patel M, Potter W. Female condom technology: New products and

regulatory issues. Contraception. 2011;**83**(4):316-321

[16] rhsc-brief-female-condom_A4.pdf [Internet]. [cited 2023 Apr 9]. Available from: https://www.rhsupplies.org/fileadmin/uploads/rhsc/Working_Groups/New_Underused_RH_Technologies_Caucus/Documents/Technical_Briefs/rhsc-brief-female-condom_A4.pdf

[17] Sanders SA, Yarber WL, Kaufman EL, Crosby RA, Graham CA, Milhausen RR, et al. Condom use errors and problems: A global view. Sexual Health. 2012;**9**(1):81-95

[18] Zirong H, Junqing W, Coffey PS, Kilbourne-Brook M, Yufeng Z, Wang C, et al. Performance of the Woman's condom among couples in Shanghai, China. The European Journal of Contraception & Reproductive Health Care. 2012;**17**(3):212-218

[19] Beksinska M, Smit J, Joanis C, Potter W. New female condoms in the pipeline. Reproductive Health Matters. 2012;**20**(40):188-196

[20] Hou LY, Qiu HY, Zhao YZ, Zeng XS, Cheng YM. A crossover comparison of two types of female condom. International Journal of Gynecology & Obstetrics. 2010;**108**(3):214-218

[21] Wang X, Liu M, Cheng Y. Acceptability of Phoenurse female condom and second-generation Femidom female condom in Chinese women: Acceptability of two kinds of female condoms. The Journal of Obstetrics and Gynaecology Research. 2016;**42**(11):1567-1574

[22] Wang X, Xi M, Zhang L, Jia L, Wang Y, Cheng Y. Awareness of female condoms and failures reported with two different types in China. International Journal of Gynecology & Obstetrics. 2015;**128**(2):152-156

[23] Beksinska M, Greener R, Kleinschmidt I, Pillay L, Maphumulo V, Smit J. A randomized noninferiority crossover controlled trial of the functional performance and safety of new female condoms: An evaluation of the velvet, Cupid2, and FC2. Contraception. 2015;**92**(3):261-267

[24] Beksinska M, Smit J, Mphili N, Greener R, Maphumulo V. The panty condom: A pilot study of the function and acceptability of an alternative female condom design. International Journal of STD & AIDS. 2019;**30**(11):1080-1086

[25] Pericoital (on demand) Contraception: Diaphragm, Cervical Cap, Spermicides, and Sponge - UpToDate [Internet]. [cited 2023 May 1]. Available from: https://www.uptodate.com/contents/pericoital-on-demand-contraception-diaphragm-cervical-cap-spermicides-and-sponge?csi=75af3245-8706-447c-8a4c-b18992d8e716&source=contentShare

[26] How to Use the Diaphragm | Follow Easy Instructions [Internet]. [cited 2023 May 1]. Available from: https://www.plannedparenthood.org/learn/birth-control/diaphragm/how-do-i-use-a-diaphragm

[27] Centers for Disease Control and Prevention. Effectiveness of Family Planning Methods [Internet]. [cited 2023 May 1]. Available from: https://www.cdc.gov/reproductivehealth/unintendedpregnancy/pdf/family-planning-methods-2014.pdf

[28] What are the Benefits & Advantages of the Diaphragm? [Internet]. [cited 2023 May 1]. Available from: https://www.plannedparenthood.org/learn/birth-control/diaphragm/what-are-the-benefits-of-diaphragms

[29] Birth Control | ACOG [Internet]. [cited 2023 May 1]. Available from: https://www.acog.org/womens-health/faqs/birth-control#:~:text=Barrier%20methods%20keep%20sperm%20from,can%20be%20bought%20in%20drugstores.

[30] contraception_report_cap_000.pdf [Internet]. [cited 2023 May 1]. Available from: https://cervicalbarriers.org/wp-content/uploads/2020/01/contraception_report_cap_000.pdf

[31] Are Cervical Caps Safe & Are They Right For Me? [Internet]. [cited 2023 May 1]. Available from: https://www.plannedparenthood.org/learn/birth-control/cervical-cap/how-safe-are-cervical-caps

[32] Venere E. On Research: New Contraceptive Gel Prevents Pregnancy and STDs. John Hopkins Gazette; 1996. p. 4

[33] Coppola JS. A new vaginal pH regulator for hormone-free. On-Demand Contraception. Nurs Womens Health. 2021;**25**(2):152-155

[34] U.S Food and Drug Administration. Phexxi US Prescribing Information [Internet]. [cited 2023 Apr 10]. Available from: https://www.accessdata.fda.gov/drugsatfda_docs/label/2020/208352s000lbl.pdf

[35] Phexxi Contraceptive Gel – Consumer Health Info | National Women's Health Network [Internet]. 2020 [cited 2023 Apr 10]. Available from: https://nwhn.org/phexxi/

[36] Thomas MA, Chappell BT, Maximos B, Culwell KR, Dart C, Howard B. A novel vaginal pH regulator: Results from the phase 3 AMPOWER contraception clinical trial. Contracept X. 2020;**2**:100031

[37] Phexxi Contraceptive Gel [Internet]. [cited 2023 May 1]. Available from: https://www.plannedparenthood.org/learn/birth-control/spermicide/phexxi

[38] TODAY® Vaginal Contraceptive Sponge [Internet]. [cited 2023 Apr 11]. Available from: https://dailymed.nlm.nih.gov/dailymed/fda/fdaDrugXsl.cfm?setid=6b4e54d7-6ba8-4400-bd52-75d112e6fe50&type=display

Section 4

Family Planning Perspectives

Chapter 7

Emergency Contraception: Literature Review, Experience in a Greek Center and Greece Used Methods

Panagiotis Tsikouras, Athanasia Hatzilazarou, Anastasia Bothou, Ethimios Oikonomou, Dimitrios Kyriakou, Athanasia Kassapi, Alexios Alexiou, John Arabatzis, Maria Georgada, Theopi Nalbanti, Natalia Sachnova, Konstantinos Nikolettos, Georgios Iatrakis and Nikolaos Nikolettos

Abstract

The sexual liberation of women can now be taken for granted, and access to information is particularly easy, but even today there is still many lack of information about contraceptive methods. No method of contraception has a 100% guaranteed result as success depends on many factors such as faithful adherence to the instructions of family planning centers, age of the woman, the frequency of the sexual act, and of course the type of contraception. Emergency contraception refers to any method of contraception used after intercourse and before implantation. It differs from the medical termination of pregnancy, which has 75–89% effectiveness and copper IUDs. Contraception is used to stop the sperm from fertilizing the egg or to stop the fertilized egg from implantation in the uterus. All contraceptive methods require educational awareness and emergency contraception should not be used as normal contraceptive treatment. It does not fall into the sphere of moral dilemmas if it is taught correctly at the levels of primary and secondary education and in the family sphere. Undoubtedly, the organization of family planning centers for women of reproductive age as well as for teenagers is deemed necessary and should become a priority of every government.

Keywords: emergency contraception, methods, safety, effectiveness, medical contraceptives, cooper IUDs

1. Introduction

Despite the existence of highly effective contraceptive methods, many pregnancies occur unplanned and the majority of them are unwanted. These pregnancies put women at increased risk of morbidity and mortality and are often artificially terminated without the necessary safety. The risk of conception after a free intercourse is about 25%, depending on the day of the menstrual cycle. Emergency contraception is the method that reduces the risk of pregnancy if administered after unprotected intercourse and before conception [1–3].

It is usually used when no contraceptive method is followed, mistakes were made in using a method or sex without consent, or rape without contraception. The conditions for spontaneous conception pregnancy include: fertile sperm in the fallopian tube, live spermatozoa up to 5 days, and eggs capable of fertilization in the uterus within 12–24 hours. Pregnancy begins when implantation is achieved. Fertile days are the 6 days preceding and including the day of ovulation [3–6]. One intercourse during this period has a 30% risk of conception, and a single unprotected intercourse in the cycle has a 25% chance of occurring on fertile days. On each day of the cycle, there is a theoretical possibility of conception and emergency contraception must be administered to each unprotected contact [1–6].

The purpose of this study is to publish the results of nine-year follow-up from the Family Planning Center of the Democritus University of Thrace and review international literature.

1.1 Contraception

Since the 1960s, the use of specific steroid oral contraceptive hormones has been shown to be effective in preventing unwanted pregnancy. Also, copper IUDs are highly effective as emergency contraception, while mifepristone is an antiprogestogen whose role in emergency contraception has been considered controversial [7].

Emergency contraception refers to an occasional method of contraception that prevents pregnancy after intercourse without or with inadequate contraceptive measures. Currently, available emergency contraception methods are the combined contraceptive pill containing ethinylestradiol and levonorgestrel (Yuzpe method), the progestogen pill, copper IUDs, and mifepristone or ulipristal acetate. The success rate of the Yuzpe method is 75%, while levonorgestrel administration prevents unwanted pregnancy in 85% of cases. As far as hormonal emergency contraception is concerned, there are no contraindications for its use, so it can be administered without hesitation. The use of a copper intrauterine coil for emergency contraception is very effective, with success rates greater than 99% [8–10].

Emergency contraception is applied and works before fertilization, so it is not an abortion. In the past and in limited cases, but even today for the same purpose, intrauterine devices are also used. Emergency contraception or the morning-after pill is the medicine that can be used after unprotected intercourse or where the contraceptive method has failed (e.g., the condom has broken) in order to prevent a possible pregnancy.

1.1.1 Indications for applying emergency contraception

Emergency contraception works by one of the following processes, depending on the stage of the cycle it is used:

By decreasing LH, it either delays or inhibits ovulation, preventing partial or total yellowing of the follicle depending on when EA (emergency contraception) is administered (**Table 1**).

It prevents the formation of the corpus luteum.

1	Missed/late doses of contraceptive pills
2	Failure to use a condom
3	Not using contraception or doubting its reliability
4	Intermittent intercourse method failure
5	After rape
6	Modes of action of emergency contraception

Table 1.
Indications for applying emergency contraception.

It causes histological or biochemical changes in the endometrium with the result that implantation is prevented.

Emergency contraception stops pregnancy before it starts. It is not an abortion, it is applied and works before the pregnancy test is positive. It is ineffective in established pregnancy, against which it has no potential for action and should not be taken [7–12].

2. Emergency contraception methods

2.1 Hormonal contraception

2.1.1 Estrogen

High doses of estrogen when administered within 72 hours of intercourse prevent pregnancy. This is an older method that is not used now.

2.1.1.1 Mechanism of action of estrogens

Alteration of the intrinsic motility of the fallopian tubes.

Inhibition of the function of the corpus luteum at the level of prostaglandins.

2.1.1.2 Endometrial changes

In the past, tablets containing a large amount of estrogen were mainly used. The method required taking two oral tablets (containing 50 μg of ethinylestradiol and 0.5 mg of norgestrel) as soon as possible after intercourse and another two tablets after 12 hours. However, nausea is a common symptom with these dosages. The total hormonal dose received in this way is less than the total dose received in a cycle with administrated oral dose (AOD), and only the absolute contraindications of AOD were usually taken into account [13–16].

2.1.1.3 Estrogen/progestogen combination

The combined contraceptive pill containing ethinylestradiol and levonorgestrel can be given for emergency contraception according to a protocol described as the Yuzpe method.

Dosage regimen: 100 μg ethinylestradiol +500 μg levonorgestrel (Yuzpe).

Taken 2 times within 12 hours and within 72 hours of contact. Pregnancy rate reduced to 2/3 (56–89%).

2.1.2 Progestogen-only preparations

2.1.2.1 Levonorgestrel

Levonorgestrel remains the first choice for patients as emergency contraception, 0 to 72 hours after unprotected intercourse.

In recent years, levonorgestrel 0.75 mg was released as an emergency contraceptive in two tablets and then in one tablet (Norlevo, Postinor, 1500 μg). This method has fewer side effects, mainly in terms of nausea and vomiting, than using contraceptive pills.

In the original packaging, the first tablet (as is generally the case in emergency contraception) was taken as early as possible after intercourse, with best effectiveness if taken within the first 12 hours. The first tablet should not be taken if the effectiveness of ulipristal acetate is greater than that of levonorgestrel [17–23].

The mechanism of action is largely unknown. However, levonorgestrel is thought to:

It suppresses ovulation, preventing fertilization.

It alters the endometrium, preventing implantation of the fertilized egg.

Dosage regimen: Levonorgestrel (LNG) 1.5 mg within the first 72 hours although there are data for action up to 120 hours. Failure has been estimated at 1.1–2% with the risk of an unwanted pregnancy being reduced to 60–93%.

Thus, it prevents a pregnancy, regardless of the phase of the cycle in which the woman is. However, if the process of implantation of the fertilized egg in the uterus has already begun, the preparation will have no effect; that is, it will not cause a miscarriage [13–16, 24–27].

2.2 Effectiveness

Levonorgestrel should be delivered as soon as feasible, ideally within 12 hours, following a sexual encounter during which measures were not followed or were unsuccessful, and no later than 72 hours (3 days) after the encounter in order to attain the method's optimum efficiency.

If taken within 24 hours of "suspected" intercourse, it is 95% effective at preventing an unwanted pregnancy.

If given within 24 to 48 hours, it is 85%, while if taken within 48 to 72 hours, it drops to 58%. Therefore, the sooner it is taken after suspected contact, the more effective it is. It can be used at any time during the cycle if contact occurs without protection.

In no case should emergency contraception replace regular methods of contraception. It should not be used on a permanent basis, but only in exceptional cases, as the repeated intake of the preparations can cause cycle disturbances due to the high hormonal load it causes.

2.3 Unwanted actions

The most common side effects that have been reported after its use are nausea in a percentage of 20%, as well as headaches or vomiting in smaller percentages. In addition, breast irritation, future ectopic pregnancy, thrombosis, and infertility may occur. In cases of vomiting less than two hours after taking the contraceptive dose, a repeat dose is recommended.

It has not been demonstrated, though, that this strategy improves contraception's efficacy. The likelihood that the vomiting was brought on by the pill's absorption is very high.

However, if vomiting prevents oral medication administration, the medication may be given vaginally.

Contraceptive tablets administered vaginally have not been proven to be successful, although it is known that the vaginal epithelium is a great receptor for steroid hormones used as contraceptives.

Atypical stomach pain, feeling exhaustion, headaches, dizziness, breast tenderness, blood spots, or vaginal bleeding are some more adverse effects [17, 28–30].

2.4 Contraindications

Other than pregnancy, using emergency contraception is not contraindicated.

Interactions with other medications.

When prescribing emergency contraception to women using rifampicin, griseofulvin, anticonvulsants, or barbiturates, many doctors choose twice the required dose. This tactic is based on observations of the pharmacokinetics of combined hormonal contraceptive pills, but there is no scientific evidence to justify its application in emergency contraception. It seems that increasing the dosage does not cause any particular side effects, apart from increasing the possibility of nausea and vomiting.

2.5 Frequency of use of hormonal emergency contraception

The use of hormonal emergency contraceptive pills should not replace the use of regular combined hormonal contraception. At the same time, pregnancy rates with the use of emergency contraception are higher compared to normal hormonal contraception. However, in cases where intercourse occurs a second time without precautions and in the same cycle the couple has already received hormonal emergency contraception once, they can use them again.

The woman should know that the use of hormonal emergency contraception does not protect her from unwanted pregnancy if she has unprotected intercourse later in the same menstrual cycle. In cycles where more than one intercourse has occurred the effectiveness of hormonal emergency contraception is affected by the time interval between taking the tablets and the first intercourse. The woman should know that if there is already a pregnancy, hormonal emergency contraception is not effective [17, 27–30].

2.6 Time of menstruation after taking the morning-after pill

Ulipristal (ellaOne, HRA Pharma) is an emergency oral contraceptive that has recently been launched on the UK market and has been licensed for use across Europe. ellaOne consists of one tablet containing 30 mg of ulipristal acetate (also known as CDB-2914 and VA2914). Ulipristal is a synthetic steroid, derived from 19-norprogesterone, and is a selective progesterone receptor modulator (SPRM), a class of tissue-selective compounds that act as complete agonists, antagonists, or partial agonists of the progesterone receptor.

Ulipristal acetate also exhibits high affinity for the glucocorticoid receptor and *in vivo* antiglucocorticoid effects have been observed in animals. However, no such effects have been observed in humans, even after repeated administration of a daily dose of 10 mg. Ulipristal acetate has little affinity for androgen receptors and no affinity for human estrogen or corticosteroid receptors [17–21].

The first SPRM, mifepristone, is used in abortions and is also an effective emergency contraceptive. A Cochrane review concluded that mifepristone is more effective than progesterone emergency contraception up to 120 hours after intercourse; however, it has not been developed for this indication in the UK and is not licensed for use as emergency contraception in no European country. It has been said that ulipristal is a second-generation SPRM. Due to variations in their active metabolites, ulipristal has substantially less antiglucocorticoid action than mifepristone *in vivo*.

The important difference of ulipristal from emergency contraceptives based on levonorgestrel is that it maintains its effectiveness for 5 days after unprotected intercourse, while the safety and tolerability of the drug have been shown to be comparable to that of levonorgestrel [17–21].

2.7 Action mechanism

The main mechanism of action of ulipristal is thought to be the prevention or delay of ovulation. A single dose has been shown to suppress the development of the dominant follicle.

Ovulation can be prevented by ulipristal administration immediately before or, in certain situations, just after the peak of luteinizing hormone. Changes in the endometrium might also be important. Administration of ulipristal during the early luteal phase results in delayed endometrial maturation and changes in progesterone-dependent markers of implantation. If given in the mid-luteal phase it has been shown to cause premature endometrial bleeding in a dose-dependent manner.

It is possible that these changes in the endometrium inhibit implantation, making it less receptive to the trophoblast. However, it is not known whether ulipristal has a direct effect on the endometrium or whether the observed changes are a result of the effect on the ovaries.

Levonorgestrel works by blocking the LH surge but does not appear to interfere with follicular rupture when taken near ovulation when intercourse is most likely to result in conception.

In contrast, ulipristal has been shown to prevent ovulation even after the LH surge has begun. This may be the reason why ulipristal remains effective up to the 5th day after contact [21–23].

2.8 Current recommendations

Ulipristal acetate is recommended as a treatment option for patients presenting between 72 and 120 hours after unprotected intercourse or failure of contraceptive measures.

2.9 Contraindications

Ulipristal acetate is contraindicated in pregnancy as data on the health of the fetus after exposure to the substance is extremely limited. If pregnancy is suspected, a pregnancy test must be performed before taking the substance.

Administration of the substance is contraindicated in people who show hypersensitivity to it or to its excipients.

Special precautions and warnings during use.

Emergency contraception is an occasional method of contraception. Data on the safety and effectiveness of repeated administration of ulipristal acetate are limited and for this reason, it is not recommended to take the substance more than once during the menstrual cycle.

It is not advised to be used in females who have a history of severe asthma that was not successfully managed by oral glucocorticoids.

Patients with renal or hepatic impairment are not advised to take the medication due to the lack of particular research that would provide dosage recommendations. Patients with hereditary problems of lactose intolerance, Lapp lactase deficiency, or glucose-galactose malabsorption should not take the medicine due to its content of lactose monohydrate [17–23].

Clinical studies on the safety and effectiveness of the drug are limited to women over 18 years of age.

Ulipristal acetate is a lipophilic compound and theoretically, despite the lack of reliable data, it is excreted in breast milk. Consequently, breastfeeding is not recommended after taking the medicine and can be safely continued after 36 hours. After the administration of the drug, the onset of menstruation may be observed a few days earlier or later than expected. In 6% of women, menstruation was observed more than 7 days earlier than expected [17–23].

In approximately 20%, a delay in onset was observed for more than 7 days, while only in 5.1%, more than 20 days.

Ulipristal acetate may have a minor or moderate effect on the ability to drive or use machines: Mild-to-moderate dizziness is common after taking: ulipristal acetate, while drowsiness and blurred vision are uncommon, and impaired attention is rarely reported [17–23, 28–30].

2.10 Interactions with other medicinal substances

Cytochrome P450, more specifically CYP3A4, breaks down ulipristal acetate *in vitro*. There has not been any specific *in vivo* drug interaction research.

Ulipristal acetate plasma concentrations may be decreased by inducers of CYP3A4 (such as rifampicin, phenytoin, phenobarbital, carbamazepine, ritonavir, and lichen planus/hypertrophic) and this may reduce the drug's effectiveness.

Therefore, their concomitant administration is not recommended. Enzyme induction wears off gradually and effects on ulipristal acetate plasma concentrations may occur even if the woman has stopped taking enzyme inducers within the previous 2–3 weeks.

Strong inhibitors of CYP3A4 (e.g., ketoconazole, itraconazole, telithromycin, clarithromycin, and nefazodone) may increase exposure to ulipristal acetate.

The clinical relevance is not known. Concomitant administration of medicinal products that increase gastric pH (proton pump inhibitors, antacids, and H2 receptor antagonists) may decrease plasma concentrations of ulipristal acetate and reduce drug efficacy.

Due to its strong affinity for the progesterone receptor, ulipristal acetate may reduce the effectiveness of progestogen-only and combined hormonal contraceptives. It is also not advised to use ulipristal acetate in conjunction with emergency contraception that contains levonorgestrel.

The study's side effects are described below. The great majority of negative side effects were mild or moderate and went away on their own.

There were no significant adverse events recorded in the study, and no patients were removed because of bad effects [17–23].

The side effects listed below are classified by frequency of occurrence. Very common (1/10) Abdominal pain Menstrual disorders.

Common (=1/100, <1/10), The following infections have been reported: Mood disorders Headache nasopharyngitis, urinary tract infection, fungal infection, bacterial vaginitis, infectious conjunctivitis, pelvic inflammatory disease Nausea - vomiting - dyspepsia menorrhagia - uterine bleeding.

Ninety-eight percent of the women who took part in the study had their next period start on schedule or within seven days of that date, while 6.1% had their period start more than seven days earlier than expected and 19.2% had their period start more than seven days later than expected. In total, 5.1% of women had a delay of at least 20 days, and 0.5% had a delay of at least 60 days from the anticipated start of menstruation. The majority of women (79%), 16.0%, reported normal blood flow, and 5.0%, increased blood flow (=1/1.000, 1/100) [17–23].

Appetite disorders, Depression—anxiety symptoms—insomnia—sexual drive disorders—irritability, Sleepiness—tremors, Hot flashes, Diarrhea—constipation—dry mouth—flatulence, Mastodynia—genital pain—uterine spasm—premenstrual syndrome—genital itching—vaginal discharge.

Rare (=1/10,000, <1/1000).

Dehydration, Impaired attention—dysgeusia—lethargy, Facial sinus congestion—cough—epistaxis—dry pharynx, Gastroesophageal Reflux—glossitis—toothache, chest discomfort—inflammation—malaise—pyrexia—thirst—chills.

3. Experience in our Greece center

The effectiveness of a single dose of 30 mg of ulipristal acetate and 1.5 mg of levonorgestrel was assessed in 90 women aged 16 to 29 years and older who presented for emergency contraception, 24–120 hours (1–5 days) after unprotected intercourse, in prospective studies conducted at the Center for Family Planning, Democritus University of Thrace, Greece, from March 2014 in 60 women.

In addition, intrauterine copper coils were used in 40 women aged 19–24 years for emergency contraception. Women with a stable cycle of 24–35 (+/−5) days, without recent use of hormonal contraception, participated. The reasons for attending the family planning center were problems with the condom (70%, 105 women), forgotten the pill (12%, 18 women), and unprotected contact (18%, 27 women).

In the main efficacy analysis, the pregnancy rate was significantly lower than what would be expected in the absence of emergency contraception (0.9% vs. 6.8%). The data showed that both ulipristal acetate and levonorgestrel prevented 99% of expected pregnancies. One pregnancy was recorded in both the levonorgestrel group and the ulipristal acetate group, while no pregnancy and no side effects were observed in the endometrial group.

3.1 Clinical studies

According to literature data, the effectiveness of the drug was maintained over time and is presented as follows:

reported pregnancy rate of 0.3% when used 48–72 hours (on day 3) after intercourse, reported pregnancy rate of 0.9% if used 72–96 hours (on day 4) and reported pregnancy rate of 1.3% when taken during the 96–120 hour period (on day 5).

During the prospective study, 16 female participants (5.0%) experienced an adverse event, most commonly headache (19.5%), nausea (12.2%), or abdominal pain (6.7%). Cycle length increased by an average of 2.8 days, while menstrual length did not change.

Limited information is available based on literature data regarding the effects of ulipristal acetate on pregnancies that are preexisting or occur despite treatment. Consequently, the use of the drug in women who are already pregnant is contraindicated.

3.2 Dosage and method of administration

As soon as feasible, but no later than 120 hours following unprotected sexual activity or the failure of any used contraceptive measures, a tablet should be given orally.

Ulipristal can be taken at any point throughout the menstrual cycle, with or without food. A second tablet should be given if vomiting develops within three hours after the first one.

It is not recommended to use it more than once per cycle, as the safety and effectiveness of repeated exposure has not been established.

The possibility of pregnancy must always be excluded before administration.

Despite the fact that after taking ulipristal it is not contraindicated to continue the usual hormonal contraception, ulipristal may reduce the contraceptive effect of this method.

Therefore, after the use of emergency contraception and until the start of the next menstruation, it is recommended that sexual intercourse be carried out using a reliable method of mechanical contraception.

The effectiveness and safety of the preparation have been established in women over 18 years of age; therefore, its use in younger ages should be done with caution.

3.3 Allocation

Ulipristal acetate is highly bound (>98%) to plasma proteins, including albumin, alpha-1-acid glycoprotein, and high-density lipoprotein.

3.4 Metabolism/excretion

Ulipristal acetate is extensively metabolized to mono-demethylated, di-demethylated, and hydroxylated metabolites. The mono-demethylated metabolite is pharmacologically active. *In vitro* data indicate that this is mainly due to CYP3A4 and to a lesser extent to CYP1A2 and CYP2D6. The terminal half-life of ulipristal acetate in plasma after a single 30 mg dose is estimated to be 32.4 ± 6.3 hours, with a mean oral clearance (CL/F) of 76.8 ± 64.0 L/hour [17–23, 28–30].

3.5 Ulipristal acetate vs. levonorgestrel comparative study

A total of 150 women participated in a comparative study (prospective randomized) between levonorgestrel 90 women and ulipristal acetate 60.

The main subject of the study was the number of pregnancies after using each method and the side effects of the two methods. The doses used were: 1.5 mg of levonogestrel and 30 mg of ulipristal acetate (once).

The participants in the study were divided into two groups. In each group, one of the two compared methods of emergency contraception was used:

Group A: Levonogestrel use (n = 90).

Group B: Use of ulipristal acetate (n = 60).

The use of medicinal substances took place in the period between three to five days (72 to 120 hours) after contact, during which no contraceptive method was used or there was a failure of it.

Ten women who:

Follow-up either was not completed. Or with unknown follow-up.

The follow-up was done 5 to 7 days after the expected menstruation.

The most frequently reported side effect in both groups was headache: In group A, there were 17 events (18.9%), and in group B, 12 events (19.3%). From this comparative study, it follows that the action of ulipristal acetate is significantly superior to that of levonorgestrel, in the period of 3 to 5 days (72 to 120 hours).

From the mentioned comparative studies and meta-analyses, it becomes clear the superiority of ulipristal acetate in the prevention of pregnancies after failed or non-use of a contraceptive method, during intercourse, after 72 to 120 hours, while in our study the corresponding results ranged at the same levels.

According to the scientific organization Planned Parenthood Federation of America, if emergency contraception methods were widely implemented in the US, at least 1.7 million unwanted pregnancies and 800,000 abortions could have been avoided. A similar picture exists in our country, where the number of abortions is very close to that of births, while many Greek women have had the experience of an abortion.

This pill contains the same active substances that are included in ordinary contraceptive pills but in different amounts. Some of them have hormones, specifically estrogen and progestinoids, while others only have progestinoids.

It is worth noting that large comparative clinical studies carried out in countries such as Great Britain demonstrate that the "morning-after pills" containing only progestinoids are more effective [17–23, 28–30].

3.6 Mifepristone (RU486)

Mifepristone was approved in Greece in 2014 for the following indications:

Medical termination of a continuing intrauterine pregnancy (for use in amenorrhea for up to 63 days when used consecutively with a prostaglandin analog).

Cervical ripening and dilatation prior to surgical pregnancy termination in the first trimester.

Induction of labor in case of intrauterine death of the fetus (for patients in whom prostaglandin or oxytocin cannot be used).

There are indications that mifepristone at a dosage of 10 mg has great effectiveness as a method of emergency contraception. Mifepristone is a well-known antiprogesterone agent that, in combination with prostaglandins, terminates pregnancy [17–23, 28–30].

3.6.1 Dosage regimen

In total, 10 mg of mifepristone has the same efficacy (1.2% failure rate) as 50 mg or 600 mg of mifepristone if given within five days.

The potency of 10 mg (RU486) does not differ from the levonorgestrel (LNG) regimen.

3.7 Action mechanism

It inhibits the growth of the dominant follicle.

It antagonizes the positive feedback of estradiol, preventing the secretory peak of LH, and inhibiting ovulation.

In a percentage (9–18%), there is a delay in the appearance of the period beyond 5 days.

Mifepristone (RU 486) also seems to have good results in preventing pregnancy after intercourse. Mifepristone, which is a progesterone antagonist, is also used as an abortion drug. When administered at the beginning of pregnancy, it acts against implantation. In experimental animals, mifepristone appeared to cause an acceleration of the fallopian tube transport of the fetus and to have a deleterious effect on the development of the fetus and its retention in the uterus. The administration of mifepristone to be done later than 72 hours after contact.

The second tablet was taken between 12 hours at the earliest and 24 hours at the latest after the first tablet. With today's single-tablet packaging, the recommendation is to take it promptly and no later than the first 72 hours after contact. Since the first twelve hours after contact is considered the best time to start the method, it could be recommended to procure some package of this type of contraception in time to be present in "case of error." Advance care for procuring hormonal EC also arises from the fact that in some countries, hormonal EC is not readily available in many pharmacies [17–23, 28–30].

Ulipristal acetate is a SPRM with a primary antiprogesterone effect. However, in some countries, despite its wide availability, there did not seem to be sufficient: information on its use at a daily dose of 5 mg for 3 months, was also used successfully in reducing fibroid size) [19–23, 31–36].

3.8 Effectiveness

The effectiveness of the method is higher the earlier after sexual intercourse, which was done without protection, the hormones are administered. For the method containing ethinylestradiol, when taken within the first 72 hours, the probability of failure ranged from 7 to 26% [33].

Using the levonogestrel method within 2 hours of contact, the failure rate is 0.4%, and every 12 hours of delay increases the probability of failure by 50% [33]. It has been estimated that with the wider use of emergency contraception, almost half of all unplanned pregnancies and abortions could be avoided [33].

3.9 Intrauterine contraceptive devices

3.9.1 Endometrial copper coils

Emergency contraception can be achieved by inserting a copper coil into the endometrial cavity within 5 days of unprotected intercourse.

The glomeruli can be inserted within 5 to 7 days after unprotected intercourse and the chance of a pregnancy is reduced to over 99%. It is indicated as a method of emergency contraception in women who have passed 120 hours and in whom hormonal emergency contraception can no longer be used.

IUD mechanism of action

a. Aseptic inflammatory reaction of the endometrium that prevents implantation of the fertilized egg (creates a hostile environment for implantation, which occurs at least 5 days after fertilization)

b. It immobilizes the sperm or prevents the movement of the sperm in the fallopian tubes.

3.10 Effectiveness

The failure rates during the first year of use are 0.7% and overall in 1 to 2 years of use, the rates are 1.4% to 1.9%. Most women can be candidates for an IUD, including those with serious medical conditions, such as hypertension, morbid obesity, diabetes mellitus, stroke, myocardial infarction, and cancer [19–23, 31–36].

The only absolute contraindication to immediate IUD placement is active cervicotida, cervical or endometrial cancer, or a uterine cavity that is insufficiently sized (6 to 9 cm deep) to accommodate the device.

The copper IUD device works as a contraceptive method by immobilizing sperm. Women using this device should check the device tapes monthly to confirm that the device is in place. They should also know that their periods will be heavier and longer in duration.

3.11 Behavioral methods

Withdrawal or intermittent intercourse is the most effective method of behavior. The male intercourse position allows the man to remove his penis from the female reproductive system before ejaculating.

For women who have recently breastfed, lactational amenorrhea is also ineffective. When the woman exclusively breastfeeds and does not menstruate for the first six months after giving birth, failure rates are 2%. After six months it is wise to use another method.

The method of calculating fertile days involves a variety of techniques to calculate dangerous days. When these days are determined, couples can practice periodic abstinence or adopt some other method of either behavior or barrier at that time. The historical rhythm method has been replaced by other methods of natural family planning such as basic day counting methods, luteinizing hormone urine tests, and estrogen predictors of ovulation [36–40].

Emergency contraception (EC) is applied in cases of sexual intercourse on the "dangerous" days (i.e., a few days before and around ovulation). If, in order to avoid pregnancy, hormonal preparations (by mouth) are used, the method is also called behavioral methods post-coital hormonal contraception or "the morning-after pill".

The method is available without a medical prescription in some countries. However, many women choose not to use the method, even when it is readily available. It is the taking of −3 contraceptive pills in a short period of time in a large quantity to avoid a possible pregnancy. EC inhibits or delays ovulation. In the past, it has been suggested that it may also affect the receptivity of the endometrium [36–40].

However, this does not appear to be the case for levonorgestrel (LG) and ulipristal acetate (OG). LG and OG also do not affect embryo implantation Other potential contraceptive mechanisms, previously advocated, include effects on corpus luteum function, cervical mucus density, and sperm, egg, or embryo transport. Negative factors in method use appear to be women's lack of knowledge and confusion about how the method works and insufficient information provided to them by doctors.

4. Discussion

Sexual intercourse is a spontaneous, pleasurable, instinctive, and physiological act. It is often unpremeditated and in many instances unprotected. Methods that aim to control the timing of pregnancy have been in use since time immemorial. Ideally, they should not interfere with the spontaneity or pleasure of the sexual act but at the same time should operate when the need arises. Numerous contraceptive techniques ranging from the primitive to the highly sophisticated have tried to achieve this goal. As yet, none has been totally successful; systemic methods of contraception aim mainly at inhibiting ovulation and need to be taken for substantial periods of time regardless of the frequency of sexual activity of the woman concerned; methods linked to coitus, that is, barriers, by their nature need planning and premeditation [32–46].

First coital encounters are notorious for being unprotected through complete omission or inadequate use of contraception. The other contraceptive emergency where backup is essential is when method failure such as condom rupture, diaphragm displacement, or pill omission (especially around the pill-free week) occurs. The emergency postcoital consultation is a suitable opportunity to introduce and discuss with the woman the different contraceptive options available, allowing her to make an informed choice.

In Greece, morals have changed rapidly in the recent decades and the new generation, adopting modern trends, is determined to control their fertility. With this in mind, the goal should be to enlighten more individualized choices of the best contraceptive method and to fundamentally change public opinion against abortion. It seems that there are so many abortions in Greece because they are seen as an easy solution, like an analysis without medical and moral dimensions [38–46].

Another difficult area is the moral and ethical implications of postcoital contraception. A couple may accept a method that works pre-fertilization but may reject a post-fertilization form of therapy. It is desirable, therefore, to discuss the mode of action of these agents with the patient beforehand. There is a general consensus that postcoital agents are contraceptive (acting postovulation but preimplantation) rather than abortifacient, but this definition has not been tested in court.

Another anxiety on the part of the medical profession is that the existing postcoital drugs can be misused as a regular rather than an emergency method of fertility control. This is unlikely to be acceptable to the patient, as the total dose of hormones taken by a sexually active woman will be much higher than a conventional contraceptive pill. In addition, the efficacy of postcoital drugs is inferior to the conventional pill. Furthermore, side effects in the form of nausea and vomiting or menstrual irregularities would make regular use of these agents unacceptable to the majority of women [41–48].

Our country has a serious genetic deficit and fortunately, it has been perceived by Greek society as a consequence of avoiding misunderstandings that reduce the value of this institution.

The family planning center is not only about contraception and population policy but about eugenics and youth sex education. According to the WHO, unsafe abortion is a "solution" for many women, including teenagers, when they have an unwanted pregnancy and cannot access services [48–52].

Obstacles that prevent a "safe" abortion can include restrictive legislation, low availability of services, high costs, "stigma," dealing with health professionals and misinformation, manipulative counseling, medically unnecessary tests, and others that delay any necessary care. In our country, unwanted pregnancy leading to abortion causes many problems for doctors, theologians, legislators, sociologists, and psychologists and problems that leave almost no person, of any social class, religion, or spirituality, untouched.

Family planning allows people to have the desired number of children and determine the spacing between pregnancies, practices that help individuals or couples avoid unwanted pregnancies, due to desired births, adjust the intervals between pregnancies, control the time of birth depending on the age of the parents, and determine the number of children in the family. Family planning allows people to make informed choices about their sexual and reproductive health [48–52]. Contraception enables the couple to decide voluntarily, responsibly, and consciously about the desired size of their family, because the size of the family should not be a matter of luck, but of choice of the couple. The use of contraceptive methods is necessary both in casual relationships and in long-term healthy relationships. In our country, the methods of contraception used are distinguished by natural methods, hormonal methods, intrauterine devices, and barrier methods.

The first full-fledged sexual encounter is crucial to women's sexual development, especially in adolescence. They have a sense of sexual fulfillment, but it also exposes them to risks if there is not adequate sex education. The most important risks may be unwanted pregnancy and accompanying problems that are often caused, such as psychological, fertility problems, interruption of the educational process, social isolation, the spread of sexually transmitted diseases (STDs), and the increasing use of alcohol and other substances related to sexual activity [48–52].

Other factors related to the early age of First Complete Sexual Contact are parents' education, parents' marital status (single or divorced parents), origin from Northern European countries, or other countries with more "open" social perceptions. These factors also influence the type of relationship (whether it was evening/casual or not), the age of the partner (whether same age or not), the type of contraception used for the first time, and the number of sexual partners.

Adolescents' knowledge and implementation of safe "sexual health" practices are influenced by factors other than individual factors such as age, gender, education, family, functional counseling-support structures, and the wider social environment.

In Greece, as a "conservative" society, the family does not easily discuss sex education issues with teenagers, and the primary health care structures that work on issues that concern young people are insufficient.

Nevertheless, it is encouraging that a large number of teenagers use prophylactic methods during sex, although their knowledge of contraception, STIs, and family planning lags behind young people from other European countries. The implementation of effective sex education programs requires the collection and evaluation of important information about the sexual life of adolescents, which will mainly be from the individual reports of the interested parties, to be anonymous, and the process that precedes the initiation of their sexual behavior.

This topic causes embarrassment to families, health professionals, government officials, civil servants, and young people themselves. Extensive efforts have been made to increase the use of contraceptive methods and, in particular, the condom, to prevent unwanted events, pregnancies, and sexually transmitted diseases. WHO classifies the "eligibility" of contraceptive methods into four categories according to their possible contraindications:

The 1st category includes the situations in which there is no restriction for the contraceptive method.

In category 2, the benefits of the contraceptive method generally outweigh the risks.

In category 3, the risks outweigh the benefits of the contraceptive method. In the 3rd category, clinical assessment and/or referral to a contraceptive specialist is required, since the method is usually not recommended except in cases where more appropriate methods are not available or they are not acceptable [40–48].

The 4th category includes the situations that involve an unacceptable health risk from the use of the contraceptive method.

The same classification is adopted by various countries and organizations (indicative: UK Medical Eligibility Criteria for Contraceptive Use [UKMEC] categories/ Faculty of Sexual & Reproductive Healthcare Clinical Guidance 2019) [40–48].

Based on the previous data, the classification of a method may vary depending on age, new pathological condition, etc. The ideal contraceptive method will prevent an unwanted pregnancy, but will also protect against sexually transmitted diseases, and have a low-risk rate high reliability, excellent tolerance predictable menstrual cycles, and additional benefits for skin hair well-being and quality of life. Emergency contraception in particular with the mechanism of action recapitulating which is the following the IUD works by preventing fertilization and implantation. This makes the IUD the most efficient postcoital contraceptive. This method seems to apply particularly to multiple coital exposures, where an IUD can be inserted with every chance of success up to 5 days after the calculated day of ovulation. Other instances where an IUD may be used are when estrogens are contraindicated, when treatment is delayed beyond 72 h, or for the multiparous patient who wishes to use the IUD as an ongoing method of contraception. It is less than ideal for the young nullipara, especially one with multiple sexual partners. In the latter case, IUD use may predispose to serious complications such as the development of pelvic inflammatory disease. The IUD may increase the risk of exacerbating quiescent PID or predispose to its development. Careful selection of patients helps reduce complications, thus encouraging the user to keep the IUD as an ongoing method of contraception. On the other hand, removal with the next menstruation may minimize the risk and be acceptable to an otherwise anxious patient [52–56].

According to our results, 90% of the women participating in our study would recommend it to their friends. There are certainly problems in assessing effectiveness, as the pregnancy rate in a cycle in the general population cannot be calculated because it is shaped by many factors.

Most work is done by showing the percentage of follicles that are canceled comparing treatment with placebo.

EC users with pills have a 5–12% risk of getting pregnant within the next year. Compared to levonorgestrel, ulipristal UPA reduces the chances of pregnancy by 75% [52–56]. Pregnancy 1.2–1.8%, probability 1.8% against 5.5% of the expected (in 941 women), Surpasses LNGEA. In cases of breastfeeding, if in partial breastfeeding there is a risk of conception from the 21st day after delivery, administration after breastfeeding is recommended, stopping breastfeeding for 8 hours of ulipristal acetate, and after taking it stop breastfeeding for 8 days. Ulipristal acetate is excreted in milk and levonogestrel has no effect [52–56].

IUD slightly has higher risk of uterine perforation during insertion (6/1000). After EA administration, the risk remains high immediately and in the future if continued without contraception.

The suitable time to discuss permanent contraception.

Sexual transmitted disease risk and appropriate laboratory testing.

Forensic examination in case of suspected rape and administration of EA and antibiotics and HIV. Rapid initiation of permanent contraception.

The availability of emergency contraception does not appear to affect the use of permanent contraception or increase risky sexual behaviors. Its availability does not appear statistically in the population to have reduced unintended pregnancies [52–57]. Women who are at risk for unwanted pregnancies frequently utilize no method or use emergency contraception late. Although it is a safe and reliable form of prevention, emergency contraception is less effective than permanent contraception. Teenage usage of EC is not medically contraindicated. The Food and Drug Administration (FDA) explained in its statement that it had approved the progestin-only method for nonprescription status that it could only be used by women 18 and older and that "Barr had not established that the projestin-only method could be used safely and effectively by young adolescents—girls 16 and younger—or EC without the professional supervision of a practitioner licensed by law to administer the drug [54–56].

The best method of effectiveness is IUD placement. The medicinal methods of EC have no contraindications and no significant side effects in all age groups. Its failure is related to the time of taking, body weight, and repeated contact without protection in the cycle. EC counseling should aim to initiate permanent contraception and protect against STIs.

It is undoubtedly necessary to organize family planning centers for teenagers and this should be a priority of every government.

The targeted intervention will provide teenagers with critical thinking, responsibility, and knowledge, with the aim of preventing unwanted pregnancy at the first sexual contact with the appropriate use of contraceptive methods, thereby reducing the risk of sexually transmitted diseases. The sexual behavior of young people is constantly changing, reflecting the times of the society in which they live and the level of education they possess. Family planning centers provide an effective sexual health service and especially help young women to have a healthy sex life without sacrificing contraceptive effectiveness.

Author details

Panagiotis Tsikouras*, Athanasia Hatzilazarou, Anastasia Bothou, Ethimios Oikonomou, Dimitrios Kyriakou, Athanasia Kassapi, Alexios Alexiou, John Arabatzis, Maria Georgada, Theopi Nalbanti, Natalia Sachnova, Konstantinos Nikolettos, Georgios Iatrakis and Nikolaos Nikolettos
Department of Obstetrics and Gynecology, Democritus University of Thrace, Greece

*Address all correspondence to: tsikouraspanagiotis@gmail.com

References

[1] Bradley SEK, Polis CB, Bankole A, Croft T. Global contraceptive failure rates: Who is Most at risk? Studies in Family Planning. 2019;**50**(1):3-24. DOI: 10.1111/sifp.12085

[2] Ponce de Leon RG, Ewerling F, Serruya SJ, Silveira MF, Sanhueza A, Moazzam A, et al. Contraceptive use in Latin America and the Caribbean with a focus on long-acting reversible contraceptives: Prevalence and inequalities in 23 countries. The Lancet Global Health. 2019;**7**(2):e227-e235. DOI: 10.1016/S2214-109X(18)30481-9

[3] Trussell J. Vaughan B Contraceptive failure, method-related discontinuation and resumption of use: results from the 1995 National Survey of Family Growth. Family Planning Perspectives. 1999;**31**(2):64-72 93

[4] Sundaram A, Vaughan B, Kost K, Bankole A, Finer L, Singh S, et al. Contraceptive Failure in the United States: Estimates from the 2006-2010 National Survey of Family Growth. Perspectives on Sexual and Reproductive Health. 2017;**49**(1):7-16. DOI: 10.1363/psrh.12017

[5] Rodriguez J, Abutouk M, Roque K, Sridhar A. Personalized contraceptive counseling: Helping women make the right choice. Open Access Journal of Contraception. 2016;**7**:89-96. DOI: 10.2147/OAJC.S81546. eCollection2016

[6] Teal S, Edelman A. Contraception selection, effectiveness, and adverse effects: A review. Journal of the American Medical Association. 2021;**326**(24):2507-2518. DOI: 10.1001/jama.2021.21392

[7] Kolanska K, Faucher P, Daraï É, Bouchard P, Chabbert-Buffet N. The history of emergency contraception. Medical Science (Paris). 2021;**37**(8-9):779-784. DOI: 10.1051/medsci/2021116

[8] Black A, Guilbert E, Costescu D, Dunn S, Fisher W, Kives S, et al. Canadian Contraception Consensus (Part 1 of 4). Society of Obstetricians and Gynaecologists of Canada. Journal of Obstetrics and Gynaecology Canada. 2015;**37**(10):936-942. DOI: 10.1016/s1701-2163(16)30033-0

[9] Black A, Guilbert E, Costescu D, Dunn S, Fisher W, Kives S, et al. Canadian Contraception Consensus (Part 2 of 4). Journal of Obstetrics and Gynaecology Canada. 2015;**37**(11):1033-1039. DOI: 10.1016/s1701-2163(16)30054-8

[10] Lauring JR, Lehman EB, Deimling TA, Legro RS, Chuang CH. Combined hormonal contraception use in reproductive-age women with contraindications to estrogen use. American Journal of Obstetrics and Gynecology. 2016;**215**(3):330.e1-330.e7. DOI: 10.1016/j.ajog.2016.03.047

[11] Judge CP, Zhao X, Sileanu FE, Mor MK, Borrero S. Medical contraindications to estrogen and contraceptive use among women veterans. American Journal of Obstetrics and Gynecology. 2018;**218**(2):234.e1-234.e9. DOI: 10.1016/j.ajog.2017.10.020

[12] Xu H, Eisenberg DL, Madden T, Secura GM, Peipert JF. Medical contraindications in women seeking combined hormonal contraception. American Journal of Obstetrics and Gynecology. 2014;**210**(3):210.e1-210.e5. DOI: 10.1016/j.ajog.2013.11.023

[13] Batur P, Bowersox N, McNamara M. Contraception: Efficacy, risks,

continuation rates, and use in high-risk women. Journal of Women's Health (2002). 2016;**25**(8):853-856. DOI: 10.1089/jwh.2016.5942

[14] Cahill EP, Kaur S. Advances in contraception research and development. Current Opinion in Obstetrics & Gynecology. 2020;**32**(6):393-398. DOI: 10.1097/GCO.0000000000000666

[15] Bahamondes L, Fernandes A, Monteiro I, Bahamondes MV. Long-acting reversible contraceptive (LARCs) methods. Best Practice & Research. Clinical Obstetrics & Gynaecology. 2020;**66**:28-40. DOI: 10.1016/j.bpobgyn.2019.12.002

[16] Grow DR, Ahmed S. New contraceptive methods. Obstetrics and Gynecology Clinics of North America. 2000;**27**(4):901-916, vii-viii. DOI: 10.1016/s0889-8545(05)70176-5

[17] Radley A, Anderson C. Emergency contraception from community pharmacies: Looking back and looking forward. BMJ Sexual & Reproductive Health. 2021;**47**(1):4-5. DOI: 10.1136/bmjsrh-2020-200767

[18] Stein RA, Deverakonda AN, Katz A, Schmidt EO. Emergency contraception: Access and challenges at times of uncertainty. American Journal of Therapeutics. 2022;**29**(5):e553-e567. DOI: 1097/MJT.0000000000001560

[19] Cleland K, Kumar B, Kakkad N, Shabazz J, Brogan NR, Gandal-Powers MK, et al. Now is the time to safeguard access to emergency contraception as abortion restrictions sweep the United States. Contraception. 2022;**114**:6-9. DOI: 10.1016/j.contraception.2022.06.008

[20] Goldstajn MS, Baldani DP, Skrgatić L, Radaković B, Vrbić H, Canić T. Ulipristal acetate in emergency contraception. Collegium Antropologicum. 2014;**38**(1):379-384

[21] Béliard A, Chabbert-Buffet N, Pintiaux A. Emergency contraception: practical guideline. Revue Médicale de Liège. 2020;**75**(12):770-774

[22] Uwanaka O, Qureshey E, Wagner SM, Gupta M, Theva M. Brown B temporal changes in Counseling for and use of emergency contraception. Obstetrics and Gynecology. 2022;**140**(6):1049-1051. DOI: 10.1097/AOG.0000000000004990

[23] Goulding AN, Bauer AE, Muddana A, Bryant AG, Stuebe AM. Provider Counseling and Women's family planning decisions in the postpartum period. Journal of Women's Health. 2020;**29**(6):847-853. DOI: 10.1089/jwh.2019.7872

[24] LaValleur J. Emergency contraception. Obstetrics and Gynecology Clinics of North America. 2000;**27**(4):817-839, vii. DOI: 10.1016/s0889-8545(05)70173-x

[25] Bullock H, Salcedo J, Lotke PS. Increasing use of long-acting reversible contraception to decrease unplanned pregnancy. Obstetrics and Gynecology Clinics of North America. 2015;**42**(4):557-567. DOI: 10.1016/j.ogc.2015.07.008

[26] Emergency contraception: Do your patients have a plan B? Obstetrics and Gynecology Clinics of North America. 2015;**42**(4):699-712. DOI: 10.1016/j.ogc.2015.08.003

[27] Nelson AL. The intrauterine contraceptive device. Obstetrics and Gynecology Clinics of North America. 2000;**27**(4):723-740. DOI: 10.1016/s0889-8545(05)70170-4

[28] Morse JE, Ramesh S, Jackson A. Reassessing unintended pregnancy: Toward a patient-centered approach to family planning. Obstetrics and Gynecology Clinics of North America. 2017;**44**(1):27-40. DOI: 10.1016/j.ogc.2016.10.003

[29] Association of Women's Health, Obstetric and Neonatal Nurses. Emergency contraception. Journal of Obstetric, Gynecologic, and Neonatal Nursing. 2017;**46**(6):886-888. DOI: 10.1016/j.jogn.2017.09.004

[30] Slomski A. Emergency contraception caution for women with obesity. Journal of the American Medical Association. 2022;**328**(4):322. DOI: 10.1001/jama.2022.12180

[31] Tyson NA. Reproductive health: Options, strategies, and empowerment of women. Obstetrics and Gynecology Clinics of North America. 2019;**46**(3):409-430. DOI: 10.1016/j.ogc.2019.04.002

[32] Khan SA, Hafeez H, Akbar R, Ayub J. Emergency contraception: An overview among users. Journal of Ayub Medical College Abbottabad. 2015;**27**(1):51-54

[33] Bastianelli C, Rosato E, Farris M, Benagiano G. Emergency contraception: a survey of 1773 women. The European Journal of Contraception & Reproductive Health Care. 2016;**21**(6):455-461. DOI: 10.1080/13625187.2016.1237630

[34] Yang C. The inequity of conscientious objection: Refusal of emergency contraception. Nursing Ethics. 2020;**27**(6):1408-1417. DOI: 10.1177/0969733020918926

[35] Montanari Vergallo G, Zaami S, Di Luca NM, Marinelli E. The conscientious objection: Debate on emergency contraception. La Clinica Terapeutica. 2017;**168**(2):e113-e119. DOI: 10.7417/CT.2017.1991

[36] Salcedo J, Cleland K, Bartz D, Thompson I. Society of Family Planning Clinical Recommendation: Emergency contraception. Contraception. 2023;**121**:109958. DOI: 10.1016/j.contraception.2023.109958

[37] Lee SC, Norman WV. Emergency contraception subsidy in Canada: A comparative policy analysis. BMC Health Services Research. 2022;**22**(1):1110. DOI: 10.1186/s12913-022-08416-1

[38] Shen J, Che Y, Showell E, Chen K, Cheng L. Interventions for emergency contraception. Cochrane Database of Systematic Reviews. 2019;**1**(1):CD001324. DOI: 10.1002/14651858.CD001324.pub6

[39] Hargrave AS, Ong A, Raza Z, Franco C, Castro AE, Nickols S, et al. Opportunities for improving provision of emergency contraception in California. Contraception. 2022;**113**:71-72. DOI: 10.1016/j.contraception.2022.03.024

[40] Zaami S, Signore F, Baffa A, Votino R, Marinelli E, Del Rio A. Emergency contraception: unresolved clinical, ethical and legal quandaries still linger. Panminerva Medica. 2021;**63**(1):75-85. DOI: 10.23736/S0031-0808.20.03921-X

[41] Cleland K, Raymond EG, Westley E, Trussell J. Emergency contraception review: Evidence-based recommendations for clinicians. Clinical Obstetrics and Gynecology. 2014;**57**(4):741-750. DOI: 10.1097/GRF.0000000000000056

[42] Lee JK, Schwarz EB. The safety of available and emerging options for emergency contraception. Expert Opinion on Drug

Safety. 2017;**16**(10):1163-1171. DOI: 10.1080/14740338.2017.1354985

[43] Shen J, Che Y, Showell E, Chen K, Cheng L. Interventions for emergency contraception. Cochrane Database of Systematic Reviews. 2017;**8**:8, CD001324. DOI: 10.1002/14651858.CD001324.pub5

[44] Gilbert AL, Hoffman BL. Contraceptive technology: Present and future. Obstetrics and Gynecology Clinics of North America. 2021;**48**(4):723-735. DOI: 10.1016/j.ogc.2021.07.001

[45] Lotke PS, Kaneshiro B. Contraception. Obstetrics and Gynecology Clinics of North America. 2015;**42**(4):xv-xvi. DOI: 10.1016/j.ogc.2015.08.005

[46] Raidoo S, Kaneshiro B. Providing contraception to adolescents. Obstetrics and Gynecology Clinics of North America. 2015;**42**(4):631-645. DOI: 10.1016/j.ogc.2015.08.004

[47] Tracy EE. Contraception: Menarche to menopause. Obstetrics and Gynecology Clinics of North America. 2017;**44**(2):143-158. DOI: 10.1016/j.ogc.2017.02.001

[48] Thaxton L, Espey E. Family planning American style redux: Unintended pregnancy improves, barriers remain. Obstetrics and Gynecology Clinics of North America. 2017;**44**(1):41-56. DOI: 10.1016/j.ogc.2016.11.001

[49] Prine L. Emergency contraception, myths and facts. Obstetrics and Gynecology Clinics of North America. 2007;**34**(1):127-136, ix-x. DOI: 10.1016/j.ogc.2007.01.004

[50] Benson LS, Micks EA. Why stop now? Extended and continuous regimens of combined hormonal contraceptive methods. Obstetrics and Gynecology Clinics of North America. 2015;**42**(4):669-681. DOI: 10.1016/j.ogc.2015.07.009

[51] Rayburn WF. Contraceptive needs--a gateway to the obstetrician-Gynecologist's office. Obstetrics and Gynecology Clinics of North America. 2015;**42**(4) xiii-xiv. DOI: 10.1016/j.ogc.2015.08.006

[52] Mittal S. Emergency contraception: Which is the best? Minerva Ginecologica. 2016;**68**(6):687-699

[53] Black KI, Hussainy SY. Emergency contraception: Oral and intrauterine options. Australian Family Physician. 2017;**46**(10):722-726

[54] Endler M, Li R, Gemzell DK. Effect of levonorgestrel emergency contraception on implantation and fertility: A review. Contraception. 2022;**109**:8-18. DOI: 10.1016/j.contraception.2022.01.006

[55] Fok WK, Blumenthal PD. Update on emergency contraception. Current Opinion in Obstetrics & Gynecology. 2016;**28**(6):522-529. DOI: 10.1097/GCO.0000000000000320

[56] Mazer-Amirshahi M, Ye P. Emergency contraception in the emergency department. The American Journal of Emergency Medicine. 2023;**63**:102-105. DOI: 10.1016/j.ajem.2022.10.034

[57] Kardos L, Magyar G, Schváb E, Luczai E. Levonorgestrel emergency contraception and bodyweight. Current Medical Research and Opinion. 2019;**35**(7):1149-1155. DOI: 10.1080/03007995.2018.1560250

Chapter 8

Family Planning and Young and Low Parity Couples: Learnings from Rural India

Priyanka Rani Garg, Leena Uppal and Sunil Mehra

Abstract

This chapter presents a research study on contraception among young and low-parity couples in India. It used the community scorecard method to understand their knowledge, attitude, perception, and use of contraception, and the barriers they face in accessing and obtaining contraceptive methods. The study also examined partner involvement and inter-spousal communication. The study reported higher awareness of FP methods among women than among men but poor knowledge of FP method availability and accessibility among both. Further, there was a positive perception of CHW's role and a high perception of barriers in terms of social norms, lack of knowledge, and limited access to services among women. A bidirectional relationship between spousal support and method satisfaction was observed. The inter-spousal communication and decision-making by women were moderately reported by women. Findings provide insights for policymakers to address family planning needs. Focusing on young couples is important due to their higher unmet need for family planning. The study emphasizes the role of men in family planning decision-making highlighting the need for improved communication between partners. In summary, this chapter presents a scientifically rigorous study on contraception among young couples in India, offering insights to address their family planning needs using robust research methods.

Keywords: family planning, young and low parity couples, male partner involvement, rural India, modern methods

1. Introduction

India's family planning program was launched in 1952 to control population growth and improve maternal and child health outcomes. The program initially focused on providing maternal and child health services, including antenatal and postnatal care, immunization, and family planning services, through a network of government-run health facilities. Over the years, the family planning program has undergone several changes in policies, strategies, and approaches to address emerging challenges and meet the evolving needs of the population. The program's key components include increasing access to contraceptive methods, promoting maternal and child health, and providing sexual and reproductive health education and counseling services.

Despite these efforts, the unmet need for family planning remains high, particularly among young and low-parity couples. According to the National Family Health Survey (NFHS-4), the percentage of unmet needs for family planning among currently married women aged 15–49 years was 12.9%, with the highest proportion of unmet needs reported among women aged 15–24 years. The unmet need for family planning is associated with several factors, including limited access to contraceptive methods, inadequate quality of family planning services, sociocultural norms and beliefs, and gender inequality.

In recent years, the Government of India has taken several initiatives to address the unmet need for family planning and improve the quality of family planning services. These initiatives include expanding the range of contraceptive methods, strengthening the delivery of family planning services through public-private partnerships, increasing the involvement of men in family planning decision-making, and promoting the use of technology and social media for family planning education and counseling. Given the high unmet need for family planning among young and low-parity couples in India, it is essential to understand their knowledge, attitudes, and perceptions of contraception and family planning services. The existing literature provides limited insights into the experiences of young couples regarding family planning, especially from a community perspective. Moreover, men's role in family planning decision-making is often overlooked in such studies, despite their significant influence on family planning outcomes. While we say this, it is important to consider an effective method that can help increase the chances of improving these outcomes.

Community Score-Card is a tool for bridging the gaps by strengthening the relationship between the community and government engagement on improving QoC. This suffices with the findings from various studies, like Ho et al. [1] analyzed the impact of community scorecards in the conflict-affected provinces of two provinces of eastern Democratic Republic of Congo where village development committee, health committee, community members and healthcare providers were the stakeholders. Blake et al. [2] analyzed a pilot intervention by Evidence for Action (E4A) programme (2011–2015) done to improve maternal and new born health services using a social accountability approach in two regions of Ghana. Gullo et al. [3] evaluated the effects of CARE's CSC in Malawi using a cluster-randomized control design. The study evaluated the effects of CARE's community score card on reproductive health outcomes including modern contraceptive use, antenatal and postnatal care service utilization, and service satisfaction. It is very evident that community score card has a direct impact on increasing the transparency and community participation in health facility management, and improving quality of care in terms of increased access to services, improving patient-provider relationships, improved performance of service providers, and improving maintenance of physical infrastructure. In addition, changes occurred through many different mechanisms including provider actions in response to information, pressure from community representatives, or supervisors; and joint action and improved collaboration by health facility committees and providers.

Judith Bruce [4] in her paper outlined quality of care standards which according to her are the neglected dimensions of family planning programme monitoring and evaluation. Hence for the community-led score card, a detailed tool was developed the taking into consideration the Judith Bruce framework of quality of care which focuses on the clients' perspectives on quality of care in family planning, service provider's self-evaluation on provision of quality of care and facility readiness.

2. Overview of family planning in India

Therefore, this study aimed to examine the knowledge, attitude, perception, and use of contraception among young and low-parity couples in India, with a particular focus on partner/husbands' involvement in family planning decision-making, using community score card method. The study also explored the perceived barriers to accessibility and availability of current contraceptive methods, providing valuable insights for policymakers and program makers to address the unmet need for family planning among this demographic group. The study used a rigorous research design to ensure scientific soundness and contribute to the existing literature on family planning in India.

The study explored the following research questions.

- What is the level of knowledge, attitude, perception, and use of contraception among young and low-parity couples in India?
- What are the perceived barriers to accessibility and availability of current contraceptive methods among this demographic group?
- What is the level of partner/husband involvement in family planning decision-making among young and low-parity couples?
- What is the level of inter-spousal communication regarding family planning among this demographic group?

The objectives of the study were:

- To assess the level of knowledge, attitude, perception, and use of contraception among young and low-parity couples in India.
- To explore the perceived barriers to accessibility and availability of current contraceptive methods among this demographic group.
- To examine the level of partner/husband involvement in family planning decision-making and inter-spousal communication regarding family planning among this demographic group.
- To provide evidence-based recommendations for policymakers and program makers to address the unmet need for family planning among young and low-parity couples in India.

India's pace of decline in childbearing throughout the country's population has been significant since the past two decades [5, 6]. The percentage decline in population growth rate was the sharpest in 1991–2001, with a decrease of 2.52 percentage points [5]. Since then, a steady decline in population growth has been continuing [5]. India witnessed a population growth rate of about 1.6 percent per year between the Census periods 2001–2011 [5]. Many states, such as Kerala, Goa, Andhra Pradesh, and Tamil Nadu, have reached the replacement level of fertility of 2.1, which was the key objective of the Population Policy of India [5]. Uttar Pradesh alone contributes to 16%

of India's population as of the 2011 census, with an average population of 199.8 million [5]. The total fertility rate of Uttar Pradesh stands at 2.4, and it is among the top five states in India where girls are married before the age of 18 years [7]. About 15.8 percent of women aged 20–24 years in the state are married before the age of 18 years [7]. Studies have indicated that Uttar Pradesh presents the biggest challenge towards meeting SDG 3.7 in terms of absolute numbers [8].

When it comes to the choice of spacing methods, traditional methods are the most accepted methods by currently married women aged 15–49 years in Uttar Pradesh compared to the country as a whole (22 percent vs. 9 percent, respectively) [8]. However, evidence suggests that greater reliance on traditional methods of family planning and low demand for modern contraception translate into lesser utilization of modern contraceptives [8]. Family planning and dropping fertility rate have far-reaching benefits that go beyond health, impacting all 17 Sustainable Development Goals (SDGs) [9].

The government of Uttar Pradesh has been working towards achieving the FP2020 goals and recently launched new methods of contraception like 'Antara' and 'Chayya' [8]. However, the state still has much ground to cover in terms of achieving the desired population and development goals, especially in promoting the nascent 'Mission Parivar Vikas' strategy [8]. The country has taken recent efforts towards addressing Quality of Care (QoC), including access to contraceptive choices, quality counseling services, information, and follow-ups [10]. Community participation has been recognized as a precondition for sustainable development, ensuring good quality care and increased use of contraceptives [11]. The unmet need for family planning among young and low-parity couples, particularly in the context of India, remains a significant challenge [12]. Despite the progress made in recent years, a substantial number of young couples in India continue to lack access to modern contraception methods or face barriers to utilizing them effectively [13]. This unmet need can have far-reaching consequences for individuals, families, and society as a whole. Unplanned and closely spaced pregnancies can lead to increased health risks for both mothers and children, contribute to population growth, strain limited resources, and impede efforts to improve the overall quality of life [14]. It is crucial to address this unmet need through targeted interventions, such as improving awareness about family planning options, expanding access to affordable and quality reproductive healthcare services, and promoting comprehensive sexuality education [15].

Studies have shown that while many young couples in India are aware of contraception, there are gaps in their understanding of the available methods, their effectiveness, and correct usage [16]. Limited knowledge often leads to misconceptions, myths, and fears about contraception, hindering its adoption.

Attitudes towards contraception vary among young couples in India. Some hold positive attitudes, recognizing the importance of family planning for personal well-being, economic stability, and maternal and child health [17]. However, cultural and social factors, such as gender norms, traditional beliefs, and pressure from families, can influence negative attitudes towards contraception and limit its use [18].

Perceptions of contraception are influenced by various factors. Cost, accessibility, privacy concerns, and fear of side effects are common barriers reported by young couples in India [19]. Misconceptions about the impact of contraception on fertility and overall health can also affect perceptions and decision-making.

The use of contraception among young couples in India remains suboptimal. Factors contributing to low utilization include limited access to quality services, inadequate counseling, lack of awareness about different methods, and sociocultural barriers [16]. Additionally, concerns about method effectiveness, side effects, and discontinuation rates contribute to inconsistent or non-use of contraception among young couples.

Efforts are being made to address these challenges. Comprehensive Sexuality Education programs are being introduced to enhance knowledge and dispel myths surrounding contraception [20]. Initiatives that improve access to affordable and quality reproductive healthcare services, including contraceptive methods, are being implemented. Furthermore, involving men as partners in family planning discussions and decision-making can positively influence contraceptive use among young couples [17]. The role of men in family planning decision-making is crucial and can significantly impact contraceptive use and reproductive choices [17]. Men's involvement and support are essential for effective family planning outcomes [19]. Engaging men in discussions and decision-making regarding contraception helps to foster a sense of shared responsibility and promotes mutual understanding and communication between partners [17]. When men are actively involved, it increases the likelihood of contraceptive use, encourages consistent and effective method use, and reduces the risk of unintended pregnancies [12, 17]. Men's support also influences women's access to reproductive healthcare services, including contraceptive methods, as they can provide financial, emotional, and logistical support [17]. By promoting positive attitudes, addressing gender norms, and involving men as partners in family planning interventions and programs, we can create an enabling environment that empowers couples to make informed choices and promotes reproductive health and well-being for both men and women [16, 17].

In conclusion, addressing the knowledge gaps, promoting positive attitudes, dispelling misconceptions, and improving access to contraception are essential for empowering young couples in India to make informed reproductive choices. By implementing comprehensive and integrated strategies, India can enhance the uptake of contraception, reduce the unmet need for family planning, and contribute to better health outcomes for individuals, families, and society as a whole.

3. Methodology

The study adopted a Score Card methodology at large, and considered two sets of respondents–the service receivers i.e. the Young and Low Parity Couples (YLPCs) and service providers/community health workers (ASHA and ANM). The beneficiaries included Young and Low Parity Couples (with 0–1 child), between the ages 18–24 years. All the community health workers from the selected villages were included in the study.

4. Sampling

A multistage-stage sampling design was used. In the first stage blocks were selected, in the second stage villages were selected and in the third stage eligible respondents from the villages were selected. Based on the sample size, the respondents were selected from the villages with the maximum density of the target population.

5. Selection of districts

The districts were selected based on a composite index developed using two indicators namely, current use of any modern contraception method and unmet need for spacing from NFHS-42015–16 data for the districts of Uttar Pradesh. For the calculation of the composite index, women in the age group of 15 to 24 were considered. There were 37 districts that presented data above the state average. From the 37 districts, two districts were selected based on the recommendation of the State government, Banda and Kaushambhi.

6. Selection of blocks and villages

Two blocks from each district were selected based on convenience. The location of the Primary Health Centre (PHC) was the base factor in selecting the blocks – one nearest to the block head quarter and the other furthest from the block head quarter. The sub-centers with the maximum population density were selected in consultation with the Medical Officer In-charge (MOIC) at the selected PHCs. All ASHAs under the selected sub-centers were asked to share the list of YLPCs with the MOICs and the sampling frame was prepared. Finally, villages with a minimum 10 YLPC couples residing in the study area were identified and selected. A total of 12 villages were selected for the study. **Figure 1** details the names of the blocks and villages selected in each study district.

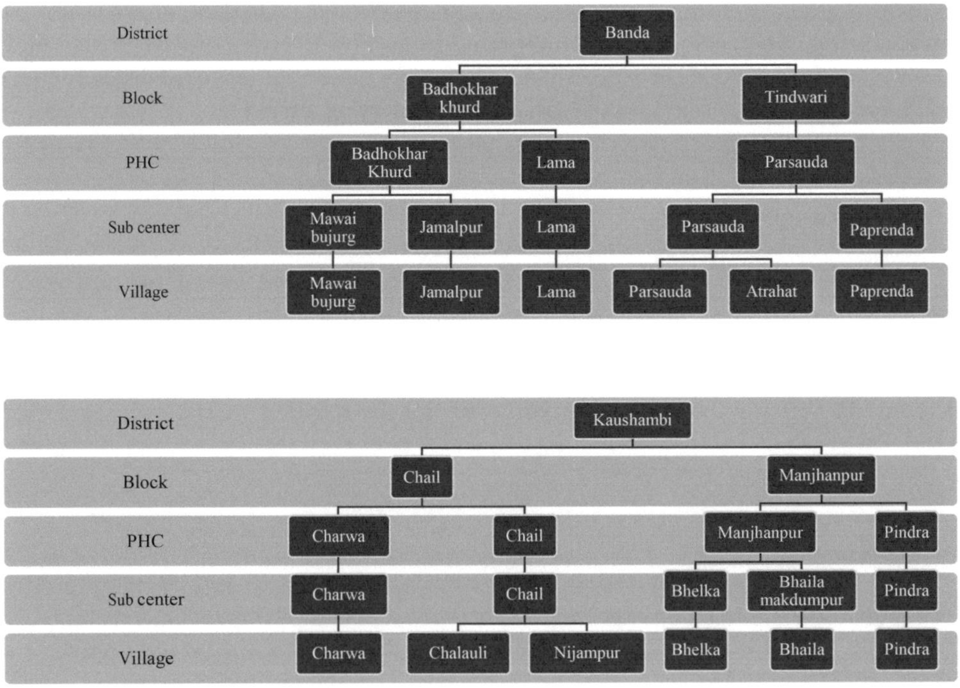

Figure 1.
Blocks and villages selected.

7. Sample size calculation

In order to determine the optimal sample size, the primary outcome of knowledge of family planning methods and services in the community was considered. Considering the assumption of 50% of the primary outcome, anticipate that the knowledge of family planning methods services in the community for young and low parity couples will increase to 15 percent point during the study duration, with 80% power, 95% confidence interval and design effect 1.2, the sample size was calculated to be 202 for each district. Therefore, a total of 404 Young Low Parity Couples i.e. 806 respondents (403 women and 403 men) were covered in the study at baseline. The sample of 30 Community Health Workers (ASHA, AWW and ANM), i.e. 15 from each district were covered under the study. **Table 1** details the respondent categories and the number of respondents.

8. Ethical considerations

Before collecting the data, informed written consent was obtained from the respondents. The data collectors explained an informed sheet prepared in Hindi language and asked for consent. Participation in the study was fully voluntary. All information gathered was kept anonymous to protect confidentiality. The ethical clearance of the study was done by Internal Review Board (IRB).

9. Data collection

The data were collected by young people within the age group 18–24 years, who were identified and trained in data collection. They were residents of the selected villages. Prior to data collection, eighteen data collectors were trained for two days by the MAMTA research team. The training program consisted of an overview of the study objectives, a briefing on the questionnaires, the sampling methodology, mock interviews, ethics, and hands-on practice in the field. Both male and female data collectors were selected from each village. The data collection was completed in 30 days.

The minimum eligibility criteria for data collectors:

- At least Matric Pass to participate as data collectors
- Able to mobilize, speak and explain in the local language and can relate to YLPC issues

Respondent Categories		Numbers	Total
YLPC Couples	Women	403	806
	Men	403	
CHW	ASHA	21	30
	ANM	7	
	AWW	2	

Table 1.
Respondents categories and number of respondents.

- Able to facilitate a group meeting/interview
- Preferably a resident of the area
- Preferably a person who has already worked in an NGO/government organization at any position

10. Quality control mechanism

The Principal Investigator (PI) and Co-Principal Investigator (Co-PI) led the quality assurance mechanism. Weekly supervisory and field support calls were conducted. Spot checks/Back checks were done. Standard quality checks before data entry (editing, scrutiny, and coding) and during data entry (like double entry, validity, range, and consistency checks) were done.

10.1 Data analysis

Statistical software CSPRO and Excel were used for data storage and analysis. The data entry was followed by the data crosscheck and data cleaning.

The Community Score Cards Scorings for YLPC (Women and Men) generated through pre-decided benchmarks framed by using results from NFHS-4 (2015–2016) for each indicator and for CHW by using results from MPV guidelines and NFHS-4 (2015–2016) {See Annexure I}. Followed by comparing the State Average based on comparable data from the same referred reports and guidelines. Each indicator is a composition of multiple variables. All indicators are on a 3-point Likert scale and they range from '0' to '2'. Positive responses on the Likert scale were recoded into '2' as a numerical value, Moderate responses were recoded into '1', and negative response was recoded into '0'. The responses were summed up to calculate the minimum and maximum scores. Subsequently, indicators are categorized into 'Green', 'Yellow', and 'Red' on the basis of the pre-decided benchmark.

Based on the pre-decided benchmark, the cut-off percentage for the highest score is decided, from which a cut-off score value is generated as the highest mean percentage score of the maximum score for each indicator which marks the 'Green' color on the CSC scorecard. A moderate cut-off percentage is decided basis of the pre-decided benchmark from which a cut-off for moderate score value is generated which marks the 'Yellow' color. Further, the percentage value below moderate is considered as the lowest value basis and the lowest score value is generated which marks the 'Red' color. For example, for indicator one, there are eight sub-indicators with a minimum (negative) response coded as '0' and a maximum (positive) response coded as '2'. After summing up the responses, the minimum score value is '0' and the maximum score value is '16' (8*2). Basis the pre-decided benchmark from NFHS-4 (2015–2016), a percentage of 90 or more should be considered as a 'positive response'. Therefore, a cut-off value of 14.4 (90% of 16) is generated as the 'positive' score which marks the 'Green' color on the CSC scorecard. Further, 45–89% marks the moderate response which means a score between 7 and 14 is considered as the 'moderate' score which marks the 'Yellow' color on the CSC scorecard. Therefore, a score below 7 is considered a 'negative/no' response which marks the 'Red' color on the CSC scorecard. Likewise, the cut-offs for all the indicators have been generated and scored on the CSC scorecard.

The facility assessment scorings were done by using the Excel spreadsheet for all the health facilities of the Village, Block and District levels.

11. Results

Scores on Community Score Card (CSC) for various indicators (eight in number) related to Family Planning among men and women in the Young and Low Parity Couples (YLPCs) are presented in **Table 2**.

Based on the responses from the YLPCs, the aggregate percentages were translated into scorecards in Green, Yellow, and Red to enable a quick visual way of their scores for the respective indicator.

Indicator	Color code	Total, N = 806	Men		Women		
		n	n	Score (%)	n	Score (%)	Score (%)
Awareness of Contraceptive methods	🟢	46	11	2.7	11	2.7	6.2
	🟡	327	154	38.2	154	38.2	42.4
	🔴	433	238	59.1	238	59.1	51.5
Knowledge of accessibility and availability of FP among YLPCs	🟢	375	237	58.8	237	58.8	40.9
	🟡	327	126	31.3	126	31.3	44.1
	🔴	104	40	9.9	40	9.9	15.0
Husband-wife communication & Decision making on ideal family size and family planning use	🟢	56	—	—	—	—	1.5
	🟡	308	—	—	—	—	83.3
	🔴	39	—	—	—	—	15.3
Role of CHW	🟢	83	64	67.4	64	67.4	77.6
	🟡	24	20	21.1	20	21.1	20.0
	🔴	13	11	11.5	11	11.5	2.4
Methods used	🟢	48	41	43.2	41	43.2	31.8
	🟡	65	49	51.5	49	51.5	60.0
	🔴	7	5	5.3	5	5.3	8.2
Support from Spouse	🟢	11					52.9
	🟡	10					29.4
	🔴	4					17.6
Hindrances in accessibility and availability in current use of contraception	🟢	31	25	26.3	25	26.3	14.3
	🟡	85	69	72.6	69	72.6	83.3
	🔴	3	1	1.1	1	1.1	2.4
Role of service provider in family planning use	🟢	434	225	55.8	225	55.8	57.9
	🟡	205	119	29.5	119	29.5	27.1
	🔴	167	59	14.6	59	14.6	15.0

n is the scores in numbers.

Table 2.
Scores on community score card (CSC) for various indicators related to family planning among men and women in the young and low parity couples (YLPCs) in the state of Uttar Pradesh.

11.1 Indicator one: awareness about family planning methods among young low parity couples

The results indicate that the overall awareness of family planning methods among young couples in the study area was relatively low. On the scorecard assessing awareness, only 5.7% of couples achieved green scores, indicating a positive response to 7 out of 8 questions. A majority of couples, 40.6%, received yellow scores, indicating a positive response to 3 to 6 out of 8 questions, while 53.7% of couples received red scores, indicating a positive response to less than 3 out of 8 questions. When comparing awareness between men and women, it was observed that women had better awareness overall. Among women, 8.7% achieved green scores compared to only 2.7% of men, and 42.9% of women achieved yellow scores compared to 38.2% of men. These results highlight the need for increased awareness and education about family planning methods among young couples.

11.2 Indicator two: knowledge of availability and accessibility of family planning services among young low parity couples

The results indicate the knowledge levels regarding the availability and accessibility of family planning (FP) services among young couples in the study area. On the scorecard assessing knowledge, 46.5% of couples achieved green scores, indicating a positive response to 8 out of 9 questions. A significant proportion of couples, 40.6%, received yellow scores, indicating a positive response to 4 to 7 out of 9 questions, while 12.9% of couples received red scores, indicating a positive response to less than 4 out of 9 questions.

In terms of gender-wise comparison, it was observed that men generally had better knowledge about the availability and accessibility of FP services compared to their female counterparts. Among men, 58.8% achieved green scores compared to only 34.2% of women. Additionally, 49.9% of women achieved yellow scores, while 15.9% achieved red scores, compared to 31.3% and 9.9% respectively for men.

The results suggest that there is a relatively balanced distribution of scores for green (46.5%) and yellow (40.6%) among the couples, indicating a moderate level of knowledge about the availability and accessibility of FP services. However, there is still room for improvement as less than 50% of couples have a good level of knowledge. Furthermore, the gender-wise comparison reveals that men generally have better knowledge than their female counterparts. These findings highlight the need to enhance knowledge and awareness regarding FP services, with a focus on reaching and educating women to improve their understanding of available resources and services.

11.3 Indicator three: interpersonal communication and decision-making among women

To assess husband-wife communication and decision-making on ideal family size and family planning use, only women were asked to score their level of discussion with their husbands regarding various topics, such as the number of children, timing of births, family planning methods, and joint decision-making. They were also asked about the influence of their parents or in-laws on these decisions and their own right to influence the use of contraception.

On the scorecard, 13.9% of women achieved green scores, indicating a positive response to 9 out of 10 questions. The majority of women, 76.4%, received yellow scores, indicating a positive response to 5 to 8 out of 10 questions, while 9.7% of women received red scores, indicating a positive response to less than 5 out of 10 questions.

The results show that overall, there is room for improvement in husband-wife communication and decision-making, as only a small proportion of women achieved green scores. The majority of women fell into the yellow score category, suggesting some level of discussion and decision-making but with space for further improvement. A smaller proportion of women received red scores, indicating limited involvement in decision-making regarding family size, timing of births, family planning methods, and joint decisions.

These findings highlight the need to enhance communication and decision-making within marital relationships to promote women's autonomy and active participation in family planning decisions. There is a scope for strengthening communication channels between husbands and wives to ensure joint decision-making and involvement of women in determining their reproductive choices.

11.4 Indicator four: role of community health workers among current users young low parity couples

To assess the role of community health workers (CHWs), the current contraceptive users among young couples were asked to score their experience with counseling about available family planning (FP) methods, clarification on FP methods, and the time provided to make decisions about contraceptive use. Out of the 403 men and 403 women interviewed, 95 men (23.6%) and 227 women (56.3%) were currently using contraceptives, and the scores on the scorecard represent the scores for these users. It is important to note that the total number of respondents differs here (95 men and 227 women) from the total number of respondents for the study (403 men and 403 women).

On the scorecard, 69.2% of couples achieved green scores, indicating a positive response to 3 or more out of 4 questions. The majority of couples, 20%, received yellow scores, indicating a positive response to 2 out of 4 questions, while 10.8% of couples received red scores, indicating a positive response to less than 2 out of 4 questions.

Overall, the results suggest that the role of CHWs in providing FP services was perceived positively by the current contraceptive users. A significant proportion of couples achieved green scores, indicating satisfactory experiences with counseling and information provision. However, there is room for improvement as a notable percentage of couples received yellow scores, suggesting that there are areas where the role of CHWs can be enhanced.

When considering gender differences, women tended to perceive the role of CHWs more positively compared to their male counterparts. A higher proportion of women achieved green scores, indicating a higher level of satisfaction, while men had a slightly higher percentage of yellow scores and red scores.

In conclusion, although the role of CHWs was generally perceived positively among current contraceptive users, there remains potential for further improvement. Efforts should be made to enhance the quality of counseling, clarification, and decision-making support provided by CHWs, ensuring that both men and women have access to accurate information and can actively participate in making informed choices about family planning.

11.5 Indicator five: methods used among current users young low parity couples

To evaluate the role of community health workers (CHWs), current contraceptive users among young couples were surveyed regarding their experiences with CHWs. They were asked to rate their interactions based on counseling about available family planning (FP) methods, clarification of FP methods, and the time given to make decisions on FP method use. Out of the 403 interviewed men and 403 women, 95 men (23.6%) and 227 women (56.3%) were currently using contraceptives, and the scores on the scorecard represent their evaluations. It's important to note that the total number of respondents for the scorecard differs from the total number of respondents for the study.

On the scorecard, 69.2% of couples achieved green scores, indicating positive responses to 3 or more out of 4 questions. Yellow scores were obtained by 20% of couples, indicating positive responses to 2 out of 4 questions, while 10.8% of couples received red scores, indicating positive responses to less than 2 out of 4 questions.

Overall, the results indicate that among current contraceptive users, 69.2% of couples perceive a positive role of CHWs based on their counseling, clarification, and decision-making support. These findings emphasize the importance of effective engagement with CHWs to ensure access to accurate information and support for FP methods.

Regarding gender differences, women generally perceive the role of CHWs more positively than men when considering the combined data for both genders. A higher proportion of women achieved green scores (76%) compared to men (67.4%). Women also had a lower proportion of yellow scores (16%) and red scores (8%) compared to men (21.1% and 11.5%, respectively).

In conclusion, the results demonstrate that among current contraceptive users, 69.2% of couples perceive a positive role of CHWs in providing counseling, clarification, and decision-making support. Gender differences exist, with women generally perceiving the role of CHWs more positively. These findings highlight the significance of CHWs in promoting informed decision-making and ensuring access to comprehensive family planning services.

11.6 Indicator six: support from spouse among current users' women

To assess the support received from spouses regarding contraception use, women who were current users of contraceptives were surveyed and asked to score their experiences. The scores on the scorecard represent the evaluations of 95 men (23.6%) and 227 women (56.3%) who were currently using contraceptives, which is different from the total number of respondents for the study (403 men and 403 women).

On the scorecard, 44% of women achieved green scores, indicating positive responses to 3 out of 3 questions. Yellow scores were obtained by 40% of women, indicating positive responses to 1 to 2 out of 3 questions, while 16% of women received red scores, indicating no positive responses to any of the 3 questions.

Overall, the results indicate a moderate level of support from spouses regarding contraception use among women. Among the current contraceptive users, 44% of women reported receiving support from their husbands, while 40% had partial support, and 16% had no support. This suggests that there is room for improvement in terms of spousal support for contraception use.

The findings suggest that women's experiences with spousal support varied, with a significant proportion reporting positive support, some reporting partial support, and a minority reporting no support. These results highlight the importance of addressing spousal involvement and support in family planning programs and interventions. Enhancing spousal support can contribute to increased contraceptive use and better reproductive health outcomes for women.

It is crucial to focus on promoting communication and understanding between couples regarding contraception, including discussing the benefits, addressing concerns, and involving husbands in the decision-making process. By providing comprehensive information, education, and support to both men and women, we can foster a supportive environment for contraception use and empower couples to make informed choices about their reproductive health.

11.7 Indicator seven: barriers to accessibility and availability in current use of contraception among young low parity couples

To assess the hindrances in the accessibility and availability of contraception, current users of contraceptives were asked to score the obstacles they faced. These hindrances included issues related to the facility providing the contraceptive method, delays in the supply of preferred contraceptive methods, shortage of preferred contraceptive methods, and the influence of social norms on family planning decisions. They were also asked to rate their satisfaction with the place where the method was provided, their experience with staff interaction at the facility, the impact of cost factors on contraceptive use, and the influence of distance to health centers from their residence.

Out of the 403 men and 403 women interviewed, 95 men (23.6%) and 227 women (56.3%) were currently using contraceptives, and their scores on the scorecard represent their responses. It's important to note that the total number of respondents for the study differs from the number of current contraceptive users.

On the scorecard, 26.1% of couples achieved green scores, indicating positive responses to 7 out of 8 questions. Yellow scores were obtained by 71.4% of couples, indicating positive responses to 3 to 6 out of 8 questions, while 2.5% of couples received red scores, indicating positive responses to less than 3 out of 8 questions.

In terms of gender, the proportion of men and women with green scores was similar (26.3% for men and 25% for women). However, more men had yellow scores (72.6%) compared to women (66.7%), and a higher proportion of women (8.3%) had red scores compared to men (1.1%).

The results indicate that both men and women face hindrances in the accessibility and availability of contraception. While the overall scorecard shows a moderate level of hindrances, women perceive slightly more barriers compared to men. The scores suggest that there is room for improvement in terms of facility quality, supply availability, social norms, cost factors, and distance to health centers.

11.8 Indicator eight: role of the service provider in family planning use among young low parity couples

To assess the role of service providers in family planning (FP) use, Young Married Women (YLPC) were asked to score various aspects related to their interaction with

ASHA/ANM/AWW. These aspects included generating awareness of FP methods, counseling on FP methods and delaying childbirth, discussing the side effects of FP methods, and providing information about the places where FP methods are available. They were also asked to rate their perception of the service providers' capacity to address contraceptive needs and suggest solutions to side effects.

On the scorecard, 53.8% of couples achieved green scores, indicating positive responses to 5 or more out of 7 questions. Yellow scores were obtained by 25.4% of couples, indicating positive responses to 2 out of 5 questions, while 20.7% of couples received red scores, indicating positive responses to less than 2 out of 7 questions. The cut-off for these scores was determined based on the percentage of respondents who answered "Yes" to the question "ever told by a health or family planning worker about other methods they could use" in the NFHS-4 survey for the state.

Gender-wise analysis reveals that women perceived the role of service providers in FP use similarly to men. The proportion of men with green scores was 55.8% compared to women with green scores at 51.9%. The proportion of men with yellow scores was 29.5% compared to women with yellow scores at 21.3%. Similarly, the proportion of men with red scores was 14.6% compared to women with red scores at 26.8%.

The results indicate that approximately half of the couples rated the role of service providers in FP use positively, achieving green scores on the scorecard. However, there is a notable difference in the perception of service providers between men and women, with men rating them more positively overall. It is important to consider these gender differences in addressing the role of service providers and their impact on FP use.

12. Discussion

The findings from this study provide valuable insights into various aspects of family planning (FP) indicators in the rural regions in the state of Uttar Pradesh, India. These findings align with global and Indian contexts, highlighting both similarities and differences in FP-related factors.

The higher awareness of FP methods among women is consistent with studies conducted globally. For example, a study in sub-Saharan Africa found that women generally had higher levels of awareness of modern contraceptive methods compared to men [21]. Similarly, in India, the National Family Health Survey (NFHS-4) reported higher awareness levels among women compared to men [22].

The study reveals that women have poor knowledge of FP method availability and accessibility. This knowledge gap mirrors findings from other studies conducted in low-income countries. For instance, a study in Ethiopia found that women lacked knowledge about the availability of FP services in their community [23]. In the Indian context, regional variations in knowledge and accessibility have been observed, indicating the need for targeted interventions (NFHS-4, [22]).

The moderate level of inter-spousal communication and decision-making reported by women in this study aligns with research conducted globally. Studies have highlighted the importance of involving both partners in FP decision-making to improve contraceptive use [24]. In the Indian context, the NFHS-4 data also reflect a moderate level of spousal communication and decision-making [22].

The positive perception of CHWs' role, especially among women in Kaushambi, resonates with studies conducted globally. CHWs play a crucial role in delivering FP information and services, particularly in resource-limited settings [25]. In India, the role of ASHAs (Accredited Social Health Activists) as CHWs has been recognized for their contributions to FP promotion and service delivery [26].

The moderate satisfaction levels reported by both men and women in this study are consistent with findings from other research. Studies have indicated that client satisfaction is influenced by factors such as method effectiveness, side effects, and ease of use [27]. However, it is worth noting that men had slightly higher satisfaction scores in this study, which may reflect their perspectives on method effectiveness and their limited involvement in method use decision-making.

The bidirectional relationship between spousal support and method satisfaction, as observed in this study, has been documented in previous research. Studies have found that spousal support positively influences contraceptive use and continuation [28]. Conversely, lack of support can lead to dissatisfaction and discontinuation of contraceptive methods. This relationship holds true both globally and in the Indian context.

The study highlights the greater perception of barriers among women compared to men. This finding aligns with studies conducted globally, which have identified barriers such as social norms, lack of knowledge, and limited access to services [21]. In the Indian context, regional variations in barriers have been documented, emphasizing the need for context-specific interventions (NFHS-4, [22]).

13. Conclusion

The findings of this study shed light on various aspects of family planning indicators in rural regions of the state of Uttar Pradesh, India. The results align with both global and Indian contexts, highlighting the importance of addressing factors such as awareness, knowledge, inter-spousal communication, role of community health workers, satisfaction with current methods, spousal support, and barriers to accessibility and availability.

To improve family planning outcomes, interventions should focus on increasing awareness of FP methods, particularly among men. Efforts are needed to bridge the knowledge gap regarding the availability and accessibility of FP services, especially among women in Banda. Promoting inter-spousal communication and decision-making can enhance contraceptive use and continuation rates. Strengthening the role of community health workers, such as ASHAs, in providing comprehensive FP services and addressing women's needs is crucial.

While overall satisfaction with current FP methods was moderate, understanding men's perspectives and involving them in method-related discussions can further enhance user satisfaction. Addressing barriers to accessibility and availability, particularly for women, is essential to ensure equitable access to FP services and methods.

Certain limitations of the study are:

- The study's findings are based on self-reported data, which may be subject to recall bias or social desirability bias.

- The study was conducted in specific regions of Kaushambi and Banda, limiting the generalizability of the findings to other contexts within India or globally.

- The study focused on heterosexual couples, excluding individuals who may have different FP needs and experiences.

- The cross-sectional nature of the study limits causal inferences and long-term trends.
- The study did not assess the impact of socioeconomic factors, cultural norms, or health system characteristics, which can influence FP indicators.

Further research is needed to explore the factors influencing FP indicators in different geographic areas and populations. Longitudinal studies and mixed-method approaches can provide a deeper understanding of the dynamic nature of FP decision-making, service utilization, and barriers faced by individuals and communities. Addressing the limitations and building upon the insights gained from this study can inform targeted interventions and policies to improve family planning outcomes and contribute to achieving national and global FP goals.

Annexure I: benchmarks for YLPCs (women and men) and CHWs.

Women

Indicators	Selected questions	Benchmark
Individual Respondent's Score in awareness of Contraceptive methods	Aware of: Condom / Nirodh	90% and above (of the total score) = Green, 45–89% = Yellow and less than 45% = Red
	Aware of: Antara (Injectable contraceptive	
	Aware of: Chhaya (Contraceptive pill -weekly)	
	Aware of: IUD	
	Aware of: Withdrawal	
	Aware of: OCP (Oral contraceptive pill)	
	Aware of: Rhythm method	
	Aware of: Sterilization	
Individual Respondent's Score in Knowledge of accessibility and availability of FP among YLPCs	Do you think that using contraceptive will be helpful to avoid unwanted pregnancy & space between pregnancies?	90% and above (of the total score) = Green, 45–89% = Yellow and less than 45% = Red
	Do you feel that young women who want to delay first child after marriage are aware of place where family planning services available locally?	
	Do you feel that young women who want to give space between first and second child are aware of place where family planning services available locally?	
	Do you feel that young women who want to delay first child after marriage are able to easily access	

Indicators	Selected questions	Benchmark
	family planning services from local public health service provider?	
	Do you feel that young women who want to give space between first and second child are able to easily access family planning services from local public health service provider?	
	Do you feel that young women who want to delay first child after marriage are able to discuss with frontline health workers (ASHA & ANM) to get advice on family planning use?	
	Do you feel that young women who want to give space between first and second child are able to discuss with frontline health workers (ASHA & ANM) to get advice on family planning use?	
	Do you feel that young women who want to delay first child after marriage are able to approach other (non-governmental) or private health service provider to get advice on family planning use?	
	Do you feel that young women who want to give space between first and second child are able to approach other (non-governmental) or private health service provider to get advice on family planning use?	
Individual Respondent's Score Husband-wife communication & Decision making on ideal family size and family planning use	Have you and your spouse ever discussed about the number of children to have?	90% and above (of the total score) = Green, 45–89% = Yellow and less than 45% = Red
	Have you and your spouse ever discussed when do you want to have your first child?	
	Do you jointly make decision with your spouse on how many children you should have?	
	Do you jointly make decision with your spouse on when to have first child after marriage?	
	Do you agree that your parents or in-laws have a say on how many children you want to have?	
	Do you agree that your parents or in-laws have a say on when to have the first child?	

Indicators	Selected questions	Benchmark
	Do you agree that your husband has final say in the number of children to have?	
	Do you agree that your husband has "final say" on when to have first child?	
	Have you and your spouse ever discussed about using family planning methods?	
	Do you agree that your parents / in-laws have the right to influence your decision on using contraception?	
Current users: Individual Respondent's Score on role of CHW	Did the health worker guide/ assist / accompany/ you to consult medical professionals to seek treatment for side effects (if any) when you informed them?	66% and above (of the total score) = Green, 33–65% = Yellow and less than 33% = Red
	Do you agree that you are given enough time to take decision on using current contraceptive method by health service providers?	
	Do you agree that you are explained of available methods of contraception by health service provider before choosing the current method?	
	Do you agree that you have clarified your doubts about the contraceptive method from the health service providers before you choose the current method?	
Current users: Individual Respondent's Score on methods used	Have you ever thought of discontinuing the current method for any reason?	90% and above (of the total score) = Green, 45–89% = Yellow and less than 45% = Red
	Have you ever regretted for using the current method for any reason?	
	Have you ever faced disruption in supply of contraceptives that you use?	
	Have you ever experienced side effects due to current use of contraceptives?	
Current users: Individual Respondent's Score on Support from Spouse	Has your husband supported and encouraged you to use contraception?	100% (of the total score) = Green, 45–99% = Yellow and less than 45% = Red
	Has your husband accompanied you to health facility centre to avail contraceptives?	

Indicators	Selected questions	Benchmark
	Has your husband accompanied you to health facilities to get treatment in case of side effects (if any)?	
Current users: Individual Respondent's Score on Hindrances in accessibility and availability in current use of contraception	Have you ever faced hindrances in accessing the place where contraceptives are available?	90% and above (of the total score) = Green, 45–89% = Yellow and less than 45% = Red
	Have you ever faced delay in supply of contraceptives from the place you avail contraceptives?	
	Have you ever faced shortage in supply of contraceptives from the place you avail contraceptives?	
	Have you ever faced hindrances due to social norms (pro-natal social norms, pregnancy expectations early in marriage, to produce multiple sons, family resistance to adopt contraceptives, lack of husband's involvement on family planning issues) in availing contraception?	
	How satisfied are you with the place of getting the method?	
	How was your experience with the staff at the place of getting methods?	
	Do you feel that cost factors / price of contraceptives act as hindrance to avail contraceptives?	
	Do you feel that distance to health centres from your residence act as hindrance to you for availing contraceptives?	
Individual Respondent's Score on Role of service provider in family planning use	Do ASHA/ANM/AWW visit your home in regular interval and generate awareness on health education especially on family planning services?	66% and above (of the total score) = Green, 33–65% = Yellow and less than 45% = Red
	Does she explain about available family planning methods for delaying first child for females?	
	Does she explain about available family planning methods for spacing?	
	Does she explain about side effects caused by contraceptive methods?	
	Does she provide information about the places you will get family planning services?	
	Are you confident that ASHA/ANM/AWW are capable of addressing your need for contraceptives?	

Indicators	Selected questions	Benchmark
	Are you confident that ASHA/ANM/ AWW are capable of finding solution to side effects (if any)?	

Men

Indicators	Selected questions	Benchmark
Individual Respondent's Score in awareness of Contraceptive methods	Aware of: Condom / Nirodh	80% and above (of the total score) = Green, 40–79% = Yellow and less than 40% = Red
	Aware of: Antara (Injectable contraceptive	
	Aware of: Chhaya (Contraceptive pill -weekly)	
	Aware of: IUD	
	Aware of: Withdrawal	
	Aware of: OCP (Oral contraceptive pill)	
	Aware of: Rhythm method	
	Aware of: Sterilization	
Individual Respondent's Score in Knowledge of accessibility and availability of FP among YLPCs	Do you think that using contraceptive will be helpful to avoid unwanted pregnancy & space between pregnancies?	80% and above (of the total score) = Green, 40–79% = Yellow and less than 40% = Red
	Do you feel that young men who want to delay first child are aware of place where family planning services are available locally?	
	Do you feel that young men who wants to give space between first and second child are aware of place where family planning services are available locally?	
	Do you feel that young couple who want to delay first child or give space between children are able to easily access family planning services from local public health service provider?	
	Do you feel that young women who wants to delay first child or give space between children are able to discuss with ASHA/ANM/AWW to get advice on family planning use?	
Current users: Individual Respondent's Score on role of CHW	Did the health worker guide/ assist / accompany/ you to consult medical professionals to seek treatment for side effects (if any) when you informed them?	66% and above (of the total score) = Green, 33–65% = Yellow and less than 33% = Red

Indicators	Selected questions	Benchmark
	Do you think that you are given enough time to take decision on using current contraceptive method by ASHA/ANM/AWW?	
	Do you think that you are explained of available methods of contraception by ASHA/ANM/AWW before choosing the current method?	
	Do you think that you have clarified your doubts about the contraceptive method from ASHA/ANM/AWW before you choose the current method?	
Current users: Individual Respondent's Score on methods used	Have you ever thought of discontinuing the current method for any reason?	90% and above (of the total score) = Green, 45–89% = Yellow and less than 45% = Red
	Have you ever regretted for using the current method for any reason?	
	Have you ever faced disruption in supply of contraceptives that you use?	
	Have you ever experienced side effects due to current use of contraceptives?	
Current users: Individual Respondent's Score on Hindrances in accessibility and availability in current use of contraception	Have you ever faced hindrances in accessing the place where contraceptives are available?	90% and above (of the total score) = Green, 45–89% = Yellow and less than 45% = Red
	Have you ever faced delay in supply of contraceptives from the place you avail contraceptives?	
	Have you ever faced shortage in supply of contraceptives from the place you avail contraceptives?	
	Have you ever faced hindrances due to social norms (pro-natal social norms, pregnancy expectations early in marriage, to produce multiple sons, family resistance to adopt contraceptives, lack of husband's involvement on family planning issues) in availing contraception?	
	How satisfied are you with the place of getting the method?	
	How was your experience with the staff at the place of getting methods?	
	Do you feel that cost factors / price of contraceptives act as hindrance to avail contraceptives?	
	Do you feel that distance to health centres from your residence act as	

Indicators	Selected questions	Benchmark
	hindrance to you for availing contraceptives?	
Individual Respondent's Score on Role of service provider in family planning use	Do ASHA/ANM/AWW visit your home in regular interval and generate awareness on health education especially on family planning services?	66% and above (of the total score) = Green, 33–65% = Yellow and less than 33% = Red
	Does she explain about available family planning methods for delaying first child for females?	
	Does she explain about available family planning methods for spacing?	
	Does she explain about side effects caused by contraceptive methods?	
	Does she provide information about the places you will get family planning services?	
	Are you confident that ASHA/ANM/AWW are capable of addressing your need for contraceptives?	
	Are you confident that ASHA/ANM/AWW are capable of finding solution to side effects (if any)?	

Author details

Priyanka Rani Garg*, Leena Uppal and Sunil Mehra
MAMTA-Health Institute for Mother and Child, Delhi, India

*Address all correspondence to: kittu.dec2007@gmail.com

References

[1] Ho LS, Labrecque G, Batonon I, Salsi V, Ratnayake R, Tran NT. Effects of a community scorecard on improving the local health system in eastern Democratic Republic of Congo: Qualitative evidence using the most significant change technique. Conflict and Health. 2015;**9**(1):27

[2] Blake C, Annorbah-Sarpei N, Bailey C, Ismaila Y, Deganus S, Bosomprah S, et al. Scorecards and social accountability for improved maternal and newborn health services: A pilot in the Ashanti and Volta regions of Ghana. International Journal of Gynaecology and Obstetrics. 2016;**135**(3):372-379

[3] Gullo S, Galavotti C, Altman L, Amin A. Review of CARE's community score card experience and evidence. Health Policy and Planning. 2017;**32**(10): 1468-1477

[4] Bruce J. Fundamental elements of the quality of care: A simple framework. Studies in Family Planning. 1990;**21**(2): 61-91

[5] Chapter 3, Census of India 2001, Series 1, India, Paper 1 of 2001

[6] James KS. India's demographic change: Opportunities and challenges. Science. 29 Jul 2011;**333**(6042): 576-580

[7] NFHS-5. National Family Health Survey Fact Sheet, Uttar Pradesh. 2020-2021. Available from: https://planning.up.nic.in/Go/SDG/Uttar_Pradesh_NFHS-5%20fact%20sheet.pdf

[8] BMC. Uttar Pradesh State Report: India's Family Planning Program. 2019. Retrieved from: https://bmcnphc.biomedcentral.com/articles/10.1186/s12960-019-0413-8

[9] Indian Journal of Medical Research. Impact of Family Planning on Achieving the Sustainable Development Goals. 2018. Retrieved from: https://www.ncbi.nlm.nih.gov/pmc/articles/PMC6183541/

[10] United Nations High Level Political Forum. Voluntary National Review 2017: India. 2017. Retrieved from: https://sustainabledevelopment.un.org/content/documents/16062India.pdf

[11] Steyn PS, Cordero JP, Gichangi P, Smit JA, Nkole T, Kiarie J, et al. Participatory approaches involving community and healthcare providers in family planning/contraceptive information and service provision: A scoping review. Reproductive Health. Dec 2016;**13**(1):1-3

[12] Singh S, Darroch JE. Adding it up: Costs and Benefits of Contraceptive Services—Estimates for 2012. Guttmacher Institute and United Nations Population Fund (UNFPA); 2012. Available from: https://www.guttmacher.org/sites/default/files/pdfs/pubs/AIU-2012-estimates.pdf

[13] International Institute for Population Sciences [IIPS], & ICF. National Family Health Survey (NFHS-5), 2019–20: India. Mumbai: IIPS; 2020

[14] Sundaram A, Vlassoff M, Bankole A, Remez L, Mugisha F, Singh S. Benefits of meeting the contraceptive needs of Ugandan women. Issues in Brief (Alan Guttmacher Institute). 2017;**2**:1-8

[15] Government of India. Family Planning Division: Annual report 2016–17. 2017. Retrieved from: https://main.mohfw.gov.in/sites/default/files/AR%20FP%202016-17.pdf

[16] Upadhyay UD, Gipson JD, Withers M, Lewis S, Ciaraldi EJ, Fraser A, et al. Women's empowerment and fertility: A review of the literature. Social Science & Medicine. 2018;**196**: 160-170. DOI: 10.1016/j.socscimed.2017.11.038

[17] Sharma V, Mohan U, Das V, Awasthi S, Gupta V. Knowledge, attitude, and practices of contraception among eligible couples in a rural area of Varanasi district. Indian journal of community medicine: official publication of Indian Association of Preventive & Social Medicine. 2018;**43**(1):36

[18] Siddiqui N, Kandpal SD, Sharma R. Community-based study on contraception awareness and utilization among currently married women aged 15–49 years in an urban resettlement colony of Delhi, India. Journal of basic and clinical reproductive sciences. 2017; **6**(2):67-71

[19] Kumar R, Singh R, Sharma A, Gupta R, Sharma M. Factors affecting contraceptive practices among married women in Haryana: A study using decision tree approach. Journal of family medicine and primary care. 2019;**8**(11):3540

[20] Jejeebhoy SJ, Santhya KG, Acharya R. Promoting sexual and reproductive health among young people in India: Emerging evidence and implications. In: Janz NK, Mercer CA, DeMartini S, editors. Global Perspectives on Sexual and Reproductive Health across the Lifecourse. Springer; 2015. pp. 3-25

[21] Cleland J, Ali MM, Shah IH. Trends in protective behavior among single vs. married young women in sub-Saharan Africa: The big picture. Reproductive Health Matters. 2014;**22**(44):17-22. DOI: 10.1016/s0968-8080(14)44753-1

[22] International Institute for Population Sciences. National Family Health Survey (NFHS-4) 2015–16: India. Mumbai, India: IIPS; 2017

[23] Bogale B, Wondafrash M, Tilahun T, Girma E, Married A. Married women's decision making power on modern contraceptive use in urban and rural southern Ethiopia. BMC Public Health. 2011;**11**(1):342. DOI: 10.1186/1471-2458-11-342

[24] Shattuck D, Kerner B, Gilles K, Hartmann M, Ng'ombe T. Encouraging contraceptive uptake by motivating men to communicate about family planning: The Malawi male motivator project. American Journal of Public Health. 2011; **101**(6):1089-1095. DOI: 10.2105/ajph.2010.300059

[25] Haines A, Sanders D, Lehmann U, Rowe AK, Lawn JE, Jan S, et al. Achieving child survival goals: Potential contribution of community health workers. The Lancet. 2007;**369**(9579): 2121-2131. DOI: 10.1016/s0140-6736(07)60325-0

[26] Saggurti N, Porwal A, RamaRao S, Raghavendra T, Ramarao S, Donta B. Effect of the ASHA program on utilization of reproductive health services: A longitudinal cohort study in Uttar Pradesh, India. BMC Health Services Research. 2018;**18**(1):615. DOI: 10.1186/s12913-018-3412-3

[27] RamaRao S, Lacuesta M, Costello M, Pangolibay B, Jones H. The link between quality of care and contraceptive use. International Family Planning Perspectives. 2003;**29**(2):76-83. DOI: 10.2307/3181065

[28] Gupta N, Bhattacharyya S, Jain RK. Factors influencing contraceptive use: A path analysis of married couples in Haryana. India. Sexual & Reproductive Healthcare. 2020;**24**:100495. DOI: 10.1016/j.srhc.2020.100495

Chapter 9

Use of Birth Control Products and Contraceptives by Adult Males: A Case Study of the Amasaman Area Council, Accra, Ghana

Hanny-Sherry Ayittey

Abstract

The study analyzed adult males' use of birth control products and contraceptives in an heterogenous community in Accra using a scientific random sampling survey of 300 persons from 39 rural, semi-rural and urban communities. The results of the analysis indicated that the respondents had no external sources of information with regards to the majority of the nine identified birth control products and contraceptives. Peers and friends were the major source of information about these products. The likelihood of using these products was significantly influenced by the extent of awareness of their availability. Increasing level of awareness of birth control products and contraceptives for men with lower levels of formal educational attainment led to their increased likelihood of using these products suggesting the important role of information about these products to socially-disadvantaged groups of people, Ever use (both present and past use) of birth control products and contraceptives was shown to be linked to higher economic welfare of respondents, particularly for men with higher family sizes.

Keywords: birth control products, contraception, family planning, Ghana, male contraceptive use, reproductive health

1. Introduction

1.1 Background

The role of men in the acceptance of reproductive health (RH) policies and the use of birth control (BC) products and contraceptives has received scant attention in the empirical literature. This scant attention on the role of men in RH care and delivery is surprising given the important role of men in heterogeneous sexual relationships which are the source of pregnancies. While women have limited biological carrying capacity in producing children, men can produce a very large number of children based on having sex with as many women as they can find for sexual relationships.

Several research workers such as Starbird et al. [1], Kriel et al. [2] and Gopal et al. [3] have drawn attention to the limited role of men incorporated in various State and

Community RH initiatives and the need to incorporate men into RH emerging programs. Men are important actors who influence both positively and negatively, the RH outcomes of society, especially those dealing with children and women. The ongoing challenge to the development and implementation of RH policies and programs is how to incorporate the role of men in family planning initiatives and the influences of men in the areas which impact the health of children and women.

The 1994 Cairo International Conference on Population Development (ICPD) Program of Action called for the inclusion of men in RH programs [4]. An underlying driver of the limited role assigned to males in the development of RH policies is the common equalization of gender with women. The exclusion of men in RH policies does not allow for the analysis and inclusion of the considerable interactions of gender with other important political economy variables such as ethnicity, race, and connections to power structures using both income and non-income measures of human well-being.

1.2 Problem statement

Ghana is an English-speaking Republic located in the western part of Africa. It gained its political independence from Great Britain on 6 March 1957 after it had been a colony for 113 years with the emergence of colonial rule in 1844 [5]. The country is classified as a lower-middle-income country with recorded per capita income of 2353 United States dollars in 2022 [6]. The population of Ghana was recorded as 30.8 million during the July 2021 national population and housing census [7]. This population is currently growing at the rate of 2.1% annually [7]. The high population growth rate imposes negative socio-economic outcomes on the country including poor sanitation and frequent occurrences of many acute diseases. Given that the population doubles every 33 years [7], there is a need for policy makers to formulate effective RH policies based on scientific evidence.

While Ghana has achieved relatively high growth rate of about five percent per year as indicated by the annual change in the gross domestic product (GDP), over the three decades of constitutional governance [8], the country is bedeviled with serious environmental-related problems which are directly linked to rapid growth of the human population [9]. These problems include extensive destruction of water bodies through illegal mining activities, rapid deforestation, among the highest in the world, and poor environmental sanitation. Another worrisome social issue is the rapidly growing national income inequality, considered to be one of the fastest growing in Africa over the last three decades [9, 10].

This research study is particularly motivated by the need to close the knowledge gaps generated from the widespread omission of men in various RH studies and also the need to ascertain the effects of culture and education on the welfare of men using BC products and contraceptives. Hence, the approach of this researcher is to establish relationships between the acceptance and use of BC products and contraceptives (dependent variable) and independent variables related to social factors such as culture and education. Given that the acceptance and use of BC products and contraceptives is influenced by the various stages of the life cycle of a human being, the Life Cycle Theory originally developed by Professor Modiglani in 1957 [11] is the analytical lens used to develop research questions.

In the reviewed literature, men were not the major focus on RH discussion. Several scholars have described this trend as worrying as males are usually ascribed the responsibilities of ensuring that family planning (FP) and RH concerns are addressed in the family [12]. In addition, national population advisory councils in many countries prioritize women in FP and RH policy formulation [13]. In developing framework for a new reproductive health paradigm, researchers have drawn attention to the absence of men from previous reproductive health initiatives and the need to incorporate men into emerging programs [14].

In light of the previous discussion, the objectives of this study were to ascertain the types of BC products and contraceptives used by adult males and to establish the factors influencing the use of these products by adult males in the Amasaman Area Council of Accra, the capital city of Ghana. Further, the linkage between the ever-use (past or current use) of these products on the welfare of the adult male respondents was analyzed using statistical analysis.

The rest of this paper is organized as follows: the next section is devoted to a summary of the review of the literature on the subject. The next section is reserved for the discussion of the methods and procedures used for the study. These include the survey administration procedures used to randomly select adult male responses and a discussion of the statistical procedures used to analyze the data. The results of the study are presented next followed by the conclusions and the list of cited references.

2. Literature review

2.1 Introduction to reproductive health and use of birth control products

Reproductive health care is the provision of basic cost-effective health services. Health services cover health promotion, prevention and maternal core issues such as safe motherhood, adolescent reproductive health. Critical to the attainment of good RH attainment and maintenance is the good quality of health services and systems in a nation state.

Over the past four decades, there has been increasing recognition that good reproductive health care could result in personal economic and social welfare of an individual (for example, refer to [3]). Despite the importance of RH decisions and practices, it is only recently that researchers have started to deeply consider RH as a key tool in advancing economic and social welfare of individuals and reducing poverty. Effective RH policies are important tools for the attainment of the 2030 Sustainable Development Goals of the United Nations for which member countries have agreed upon.

2.2 Factors influencing the use of BC products and contraceptives

The reviewed literature indicates that there are several socio-economic and cultural factors which are responsible for the use of BC products and contraceptives. These factors include marital status, formal educational attainment, culture and awareness of these products. Marital status influences the use of contraceptives among people.

Sedgh et al. [15] suggested that that the individual marital status was an important factor influencing his/her use of BC products and contraceptives. However, culture, religion and other socio-demographic factors, such as age and educational attainment, were also important drivers of the use of contraceptives.

Education and one's educational level have a relationship with contraceptive use. Women with higher levels of education are able to make better and informed decisions regarding contraceptives [16].

Cultural factors are cited reasons for the low levels of acceptance and use of reproductive health and family planning services in many countries arising from the pro-natural beliefs of adherents of religious faiths such as Islam and Roman Catholic Christianity (for example, refer to [17]). The location of a person and his/her adoption and use of BC products has been reported in the literature (Hawkes and Hart [18]). Persons living in urban localities tend to use BC products more intensively than those in rural localities arising from the relatively higher levels of education and incomes of the latter group of people. Further, access to these products tends to be relatively limited in rural areas.

Awareness of BC products and contraceptives has been shown to be a major factor driving the uptake of these products in parts of the developing world [19]. The important role of the mass media in disseminating information about BC products is weaker in rural areas of many developing countries due to the limited access of rural people to electricity and related infrastructural facilities.

3. Methodology and procedures used in the study

3.1 Survey methods and administration

The survey of adult males was undertaken in the Amasaman Area Council in the Greater Accra Region of Ghana. It involved randomly selected males who were 18 years of age and above. The period of the survey was November and December 2019. Random sampling procedures which involved confidential interviews were used to elicit information from adult householders who were male from all 39 communities of the Amasaman Area Council. Using statistical theory and concepts indicated by scholars (e.g., refer to [20–22]), the optimal sample size was determined as 292. The previous pilot survey conducted earlier in June 2019 confirmed that the probability of an adult male being aware of at least one BC product was 0.95. Given that the research allowed for 0.025 maximum standard error (MSE) to be achieved with 95 percent confidence level (that is 1.96 standard errors from a normal distribution), 292 was derived as the optimal sample size. This sample size was increased to 300 leading to an oversampling of eight respondents.

3.2 Model of use of BC products and contraceptives

A binary logit regression analysis was undertaken to determine socio-economic characteristics of the male respondents that significantly influenced the decision to currently use any of the nine identified BC products and contraceptives. The binary logit model is discussed by Gujarati [23]. The specific model used in this study was as follows:

$$\begin{aligned} \text{LOG}\,(\text{PROBUSEBCP}/(1-\text{PROBUSEBCP})) = \text{f}(&\text{MALEAGE, MALEEDU,} \\ &\text{SPOUSEEDU, MALEEDU}^{*}\text{SPOUSEEDU, PINCOMEM,} \\ &\text{BCPAWARENESS, BCPAWARENESS}^{*}\text{MALEEDU}) \end{aligned} \tag{1}$$

where PROBUSEBCP was the dependent variable expressing the probability of the male respondent currently using one or more of the nine identified BC products and contraceptives.

MALEAGE was the age of the male householder.

MALEEDU was the level of formal educational attainment of the householder in years.

SPOUSEDU was the level of formal educational attainment of the male householder's spouse.

MALEEDU*SPOUSEEDU was the interaction variable combining MALEEDU and SPOUSEEDU.

PINCOMEM was the average income of the male householder per month.

BCPAWARENESS was the average degree of awareness indicated by the male householder for each of the nine BC products and contraceptives. The Likert scale was used for the assessment of the degree of awareness with zero indicating total lack of awareness, and 5 for the highest level of awareness.

BCPAWARENESS*MALEEDU.

Eq. 2 represents the specific model used for the analysis and was based on the dependent variable being the natural logarithm of the odds ratio of the respondent using any one of the nine BC products:

LOG (PROBUSEBCP)/(1 − PROBUSEBCP).

$$\begin{aligned} &\mathrm{LOG\,(PROBUSEBCP)/(1-PROBUSEBCP)} \\ &\quad = A_0 + A_1\,\mathrm{MALEAGE} + A_2\,\mathrm{MALEEDU} + A_3\,\mathrm{SPOUSEEDU} \\ &\qquad + A_4\,\mathrm{MALEEDU^*SPOUSEEDU} + A_5\,\mathrm{PINCOMEM} + A_6\,\mathrm{BCPWARENESS} \\ &\qquad + A_7\,\mathrm{BCPAWARENESS^*MALEEDU} + U \end{aligned} \tag{2}$$

Where A_i (i = 0, 1, 2, 3, 4, 5, 6 and 7) are the parameters and U is the equation error term.

3.3 Model linking economic welfare of male respondents and their ever-use of BC products

A multiple regression model analysis was used to ascertain the relationship between personal empowerment, indicated by personal income adjusted for by household size, and the use of birth control methods and other socio-economic characteristics of the 300 male respondents (household heads). The model used is specified as Eq. (3) below:

$$\begin{aligned} \mathrm{LPINCOMEM} = {} & E_0 + E_1\,\mathrm{MALEAGE} + E_2\,\mathrm{MALEAGESQUARED} \\ & + E_3\,\mathrm{MALEEDUSSS} + E_4\,\mathrm{CUMARRIED} + E_5\,\mathrm{ISLAMREL} \\ & + E_6\,\mathrm{HSIZELARGE} + E_7\,\mathrm{EVERUSEDBCP} \\ & + E_8\,\mathrm{HSIZELARGE^*EVERUSEDBCP} + Z_i \end{aligned} \tag{3}$$

where LPINCOMEM was the natural logarithm of the average income earned by the householder per month, adjusted for by the size of his household (HHSIZE), to derive adult-equivalent income. This adjusted household size (λ derivation was based on the equation λ = (HHSIZE)$^{\sigma}$ with σ being the scale parameter. The scale parameter used was 0.70 similar to the work of Buse & Salathe [24].

AGE is the age of the male respondent in years.

MALEAGESQUARED is the square of MALEAGE. This variable is incorporated in the model to examine the possibility of a curvilinear relationship between economic welfare of the male respondent and his age over time; this specification is driven by the life cycle theory employed for this study. Hence, the linear versions are used for the analysis.

MALEEDUSSS is a dummy variable with the value 1 for male respondents who completed senior secondary school or its equivalent and zero otherwise. Rather than using formal educational attainment (MALEEDU), the use of MALEEDUSSS dummy variable was due to the fact that MALEEDU was directly related to the use of BC products. MALEEDUSSS therefore served as an instrumental variable for MALEEDU to avoid the problem of endogeneity in the regression model.

ISLAMRELIGION is a dummy variable taking the value of 1 if the male respondent is a Muslim and zero if the respondent is not a Muslim.

CUMARRIED is a dummy variable taking the value of 1 if the male respondent was married at the time of the survey in November/December 2019, and zero if the respondent was not married at that time.

HSIZELARGE is a dummy variable with a value of 1 if the nominal household size is three or more, and zero if the nominal household size is less than three (that is single-person family or two-person family). The choice of three as the threshold household size was based on a numerical simulation analysis of household sizes from 1 to 17.

EVERUSEDBCP carried a value of 1 if the male respondent had ever used BC products during his lifetime. It took a value of zero if the respondent had never used any BC products in his lifetime.

HHSIZELARGE*EVERUSEDBCP is an interaction term between the two variables, HHSIZELARGE and EVERUSEDBCP, that evaluates the effect of the use of BC products in larger-sized households of three or more on the economic welfare of the male respondent. Larger-sized households used in this study indicate that the household has an adult male with a spouse and at least one dependent.

E_i (where i = 0,1,2,3,4,5,6 and 7) are parameters to be estimated; and Z is the equation error term, initially assumed to have zero mean and constant variance.

4. Results

The socio-economic characteristics of these 300 respondents, based on frequency analysis, are presented in **Table 1**. The age range of the respondents was between 20 and 69. However, the dominant age group of the respondents was the 30 to 49 years group; this group had about three-quarters of all the respondents (77.7%). The vast majority of the respondents has some formal schooling with only 4.6% never attending school. About two-thirds of the respondents were formally married (66.9%) while about one quarter were in various cohabitation arrangements with partners ((26.2%).

In terms of religious affiliation, Christianity was declared as the dominant religion with over three-quarters (76.8%) of the respondents indicating this religion as their preference. Following Christianity, the most popular religious affiliation was traditional African religions, either in their sole forms or mixed with Christianity or Islam;

Item/ group	Percentage (%)
Age group	
20–29	18.2
30–39	54.3
40–49	25.2
50–59	2.0
60–69	0.3
Educational level	
No schooling	4.6
Primary school	3.6
Junior high school/Middle School	19.9
Some senior high school	13.9
Senior high school graduate	18.2
Post-junior high school technical school	0.0
Technical college/school	19.2
Higher National Diploma Holder	13.2
Diploma	5.6
Bachelor degree holder	1.0
Postgraduate degree holder	0.7
Religious Affiliation	
Christian Protestant	36.4
Christian Roman Catholic	23.8
Christian Charismatic or Pentecostal	14.9
Christian Jehovah Witnesses	0.0
Christian/African traditionalist	7.3
Islam	7.3
Islam/African traditionalist	2.3
Traditional African religions adherents	4.6
Atheist	0.7
Buddhism	0.7
Hare Krishna	0.3
Ethnicity (Broad Ethnic Group)	
Akan	20.5
Dangme/Ga	17.5
Ewe	31.8
Guan	12.6
Gurma	6.0
Mole-Dagbani	3.6
Grusi	2.7
Mande	0.6
All Other groups	2.3
Occupation	
Self- employed/own business	29.1
Private sector employee	20.9
Government sector employee	7.3
Artisans	30.1
Farmers	11.6
Unemployed	1.0
Marital Status	
Currently Married	66.9
Cohabitation	26.2
Divorced	3.3

Item/ group	Percentage (%)
Widowed	1.3
Single	2.4
Membership of Community Associations, Groups and Organizations	
No association	0.0
Political Parties	56.9
Men Fellowship (Christian)	10.6
Islamic Brotherhood/Political Parties	7.6
Men Fellowship/Political Parties	22.2
Current Use of Birth Control Methods (Within the Last 12 Months Before Survey)	
Yes	13.9
No	86.1
Past Use of Birth Control Methods (Beyond the Last 12 Months Prior to the Survey)	
Yes	14.9
No	85.1
Current Use of Birth Control Methods by the Spouse of the Respondent (Within the Last 12 Months Before Survey)	
Yes	19.2
No	46.7
Respondent Does Not Know	34.1

Source: Data from survey undertaken in November and December 2019.

Table 1.
Characteristics of the male survey respondents based on frequency analysis.

this mixed preference was indicated by about one in seven of the respondents (14.2%). Ghana has nine broad ethnic groups. The largest ethnic group among the respondents was Ewe. The second largest group was Akan and this was followed by Dangme/Ga groups.

In terms of employment, artisans were the largest group followed by self-employed people from other categories and then by private sector employees, farmers and government sector employees. With regards to the use of BC products, about one in seven of the respondents (13.9%) had used these products during the 12 months before the start of the survey. This proportion was slightly smaller than the proportion of the respondents who had used these products during past periods (14.9%).

Table 2 represents the summary socio-economic characteristics in terms of average or mean figures. The average age was 35.6 years, ranging from 22 to 60 years. The number of years of formal schooling acquired was 11.0 years. The average number of people living in a household was 6.0 and the average number of children was 3.8, 2.1 male children and 1.7 female children. The average monthly income received by the adult male was about 499 Ghana cedis during the year, 2019. Given that one United States dollar was worth on average 5.22 Ghana cedis in 2019, the average monthly income translated to about 96 US dollars. The amount of money spent on BC products and contraceptives, over the previous year, was 24 Ghana cedis or about 4.6 United States dollars.

As indicated in the literature, the quality attributes of available and accessible health services and systems influences the use of BC products and contraceptives. **Table 3** contains the scores for the various quality attributes of health services and health systems declared by the respondents. The lowest-ranked service or facility was

Item	Mean	SD	Range
Age in years	35.6	6.0	22 to 60
Total personal income of respondents per month, Ghana Cedis (GHC)	498.8	203.2	0 to 1450
Number of years of formal schooling	11.0	3.3	0 to 18
Number of people in the household	6.0	1.7	2 to 17
Expenditures on BC products during the previous 12 months	24.0	59.7	0 to 400
Source: Data from survey undertaken in November and December 2019.			

Table 2.
Summary of characteristics of male survey respondents based on averages.

the sanitary condition of the facility. The average quality score for this attribute was 1.705. On the other hand, the highest ranked attribute was the ease of access to the health centre or clinic with an average score of 4.301 out of the maximum score of 5.0. Services provided by doctors at the health centre or clinic were generally considered to be in the very good to excellent range and further the quality values exceeded those indicated for services provided by nurses and pharmacists (refer to **Table 3**). The quality of services provided by pharmacists and nurses at the health centre and clinic

Item	Number	Average Score	Standard Deviation	Ranking
Health Centre or Clinic				
Distance to the Health Centre or Clinic	300	3.768	0.845	3
Time to the Health Centre or Clinic	300	3.884	0.731	2
Ease of Access to the Facility on Arrival	300	4.301	0.587	1
Availability of Comfortable Seating Arrangements	300	3.020	0.896	4
Availability of Toilet and Urinary Facilities	300	1.705	0.712	5
Health Centre (Nurses)				
Knowledge of my health condition	227	3.634	0.766	1
Willingness to help treat my health condition	227	3.546	0.946	2
Provision of information concerning my health condition	227	2.705	0.870	4
Level of friendliness and care from personnel	227	2.661	0.970	5
Overall usefulness of interaction with Nurse(s)	227	3.537	0.827	3
Health Personnel (Pharmacists)				
Knowledge of my health condition	163	2.663	0.678	4
Willingness to help treat my health condition	163	2.798	0.721	2
Provision of information concerning my health condition	163	2.558	0.658	5
Level of friendliness and care from personnel	163	2.712	0.767	3
Overall usefulness of interaction with Pharmacist(s)	161	3.248	0.994	1

Item	Number	Average Score	Standard Deviation	Ranking
Health Personnel (Doctors)				
Knowledge of my health condition	184	4.636	0.483	1
Willingness to help treat my health condition	246	4.550	0.545	3
Provision of information concerning my health condition	246	4.386	0.627	5
Level of friendliness and care from personnel	246	4.463	0.583	4

The assessment of the quality of services or access to services that you received at the health centre that you last visited based a Likert scale of 0 to 5 denoting excellent quality, 4 very good quality, 3 moderate quality, 2 low quality, 1 very low quality and zero (0) for no quality at all. Source: Data from survey undertaken in November and December 2019.

Table 3.
Quality assessment scores of health services and systems by respondents.

was generally similar; however the average quality scores were slightly higher for services provided by nurses.

The study identified nine BC products and methods which were known by the male respondents. These are reported in **Table 4**. The traditional method of planned abstinence from the spouse for a period of time, after the delivery of a child was the most familiar BC method or product. Male condom was the second most important BC method or product. Other BC methods and products identified by the male respondents were vasectomy, rhythm or calendar method, traditional herbs, outercourse, drinking of local gin before sex, and taking drugs to prevent pregnancy.

Table 5 shows the most important single sources of information for the BC methods and products. There were no source of awareness for five BC methods and

No.	Method	No.	Average score of importance	Standard deviation of score	Ranking
1	Traditional method - planned abstinence	300	4.470	0.629	1
2	Male condom	300	3.917	1.036	2
3	Withdrawal before ejaculation	300	3.076	1.291	3
4	Vasectomy (male sterilization)	300	1.328	1.016	4
5	Rhythm or calendar method of the woman's monthly reproductive cycle	300	0.940	0.931	5
6	Traditional herbs	300	0.887	1.147	6
7	Outercourse (sex without penetration)	300	0.626	0.817	7
8	Drinking of local gin before sex	300	0.606	0.926	8
9	Men taking drugs to prevent pregnancy	300	0.447	0.688	9

The scoring is based on 5 denoting that item is very high level of awareness, 4 represented high level of awareness, 3 indicated moderate level of awareness, 2 represented low level of awareness, 1 represented very low level of awareness and zero (0) represented total lack of awareness of the particular birth control method. The coefficient of variation is the standard deviation divided by the mean score. Source: Data from survey undertaken in November and December 2019.

Table 4.
Ranking of the level of awareness of birth control methods by respondents.

Item	Type of Birth Control Method	Most Important Source of Information	Percent of Respondents
1	Traditional method - planned abstinence	Information obtained from parents, carers and other relatives	52.6
2	Male condom	Advertisement through television	32.5
3	Withdrawal before ejaculation	Information from peers and friends	59.6
4	Vasectomy (male sterilization)	Information from peers and friends	38.7
5	Rhythm or calendar	No source of awareness	35.8
6	Traditional herbs	No source of awareness	52.3
7	Outercourse (sex without penetration)	No source of awareness	53.6
8	Drinking of local gin before sex	No source of awareness	62.3
9	Men taking drugs to prevent pregnancy	No source of awareness	65.9

Source: Data from survey undertaken in November and December 2019.

Table 5.
The most important source of information for various birth control methods as declared by the respondents.

products. These were rhythm method, traditional herbs, outercourse, drinking of local gin before sex, and taking drugs to prevent pregnancy. Further, peers and friends were the most source of information for the BC methods and products: withdrawal before ejaculation and vasectomy. Television was the major source of information for the male condom. This result on male condom was also established by Anaman and Okai [25], for females.

The intensity of the use of BC methods and products is summarized in **Tables 6** and 7. **Table 6** provides information on the use intensity during the previous 12 months before the survey, considered to refer to current use. The information in **Table 7** refers to past use intensity of the various BC methods and products. The commonest BC method or product was the male condom. Withdrawal before ejaculation was the second most important BC method or product. The findings of

Item	Method	No.	Average score of importance	Standard deviation of score	Ranking
1	Traditional method - planned abstinence	10	0.900	1.912	3
2	Male condom	34	2.853	1.019	1
3	Withdrawal before ejaculation	10	1.20	1.619	2
4	Vasectomy (male sterilization)	9	0.56	1.667	4
5	Rhythm or calendar	8	0.00	0.00	7
6	Traditional herbs	10	0.40	0.843	6
7	Outercourse (sex without penetration)	9	0.00	0.00	7
8	Drinking of local gin before sex	8	0.00	0.00	7

Item	Method	No.	Average score of importance	Standard deviation of score	Ranking
9	Men taking drugs to prevent pregnancy	9	0.556	1.667	5

The scoring is based on 5 denoting that item is very high level of use, 4 represented high level of use, 3 indicated moderate level of use, 2 represented low level of use, 1 represented very low level of use, and zero (0) represented total lack of use of the particular birth control method. The coefficient of variation is the standard deviation divided by the mean score. Source: Data from survey undertaken in November and December 2019.

Table 6.
Ranking of the level of intensity of current use of birth control methods by respondents.

No.	Method	No.	Average score of importance	Standard deviation of score	Ranking
1	Traditional method - planned abstinence	12	0.750	1.765	2
2	Male condom	37	2.973	0.897	1
3	Withdrawal before ejaculation	10	0.00	0.00	6
4	Vasectomy (male sterilization)	11	0.45	1.508	5
5	Rhythm or calendar	10	0.00	0.00	6
6	Traditional herbs	14	0.64	1.151	3
7	Outercourse (sex without penetration)	10	0.00	0.00	6
8	Drinking of local gin before sex	10	0.00	0.00	6
9	Men taking drugs to prevent pregnancy	12	0.583	1.505	4

The scoring is based on 5 denoting that item is very high level of use, 4 represented high level of use, 3 indicated moderate level of use, 2 represented low level of use, 1 represented very low level of use, and zero (0) represented total lack of use of the particular birth control method. The coefficient of variation is the standard deviation divided by the mean score. Source: Derived from survey data, November to December 2019.

Table 7.
Ranking of the level of intensity of past use of birth control methods by male respondents.

this study corroborate the disconnect between the awareness of BC methods and products and their relatively low intensity of use in Ghana established by other studies such as [26, 27].

Table 8 provides the reasons given by the respondents for *not currently using* BC methods and products. The assertion that BC methods and products were meant for women and not men was the most important reasons given by the male respondents for their non-use of these products during the current period (within 12 months of the survey). The dislike of the BC methods and products was cited as the second most important reason for their non-use by the male respondents. The third most important reason was the perceived harmful side effects from the use of these products.

Table 9 summarizes the suggested reasons for non-use of BC methods and products during the past periods. The results assembled in **Table 9** are similar to those reported in **Table 8** with very close figures for the percentages of the male respondents expressing similar sentiments with regards to the three most important reasons

Reason for not using BC products	% of respondents	Importance ranking
Birth control methods are for women to use	31.8	1
Respondent does not like birth control methods	23.8	2
Use of birth control methods can cause serious side effects	10.3	3
Use of control methods is against cultural beliefs	9.2	4
Birth control products are not readily available	9.2	5
Birth control products are very expensive	8.0	6
Use of birth control methods is against religious beliefs	6.5	7
Birth control methods can use male or female infertility	1.1	8

Source: Data from survey undertaken in November and December 2019.

Table 8.
Reasons given by the male respondents for not currently using birth control methods and products based on the percentage of respondents.

Reason for not using birth control methods	Respondents declaring this reason (%)	Ranking
Birth control methods are for women to use	31.2	1
Respondent does not like birth control methods	23.8	2
Birth control products are not readily available	11.2	3
Birth control products are very expensive	9.6	4
Use of birth control methods is against religious beliefs	8.1	5
Use of birth control methods can cause serious side effects	7.7	6
Use of control methods is against cultural beliefs	6.9	7
Birth control methods can use male or female infertility	1.2	8

Source: Data from survey undertaken in November and December 2019.

Table 9.
Reasons given by the male respondents for not using birth control methods and products during the past based on the percentage of respondents.

for non-use of BC methods and products. Non-use of BC methods and products for religious and cultural reasons were cited by the respondents in both **Tables 8** and **9**. However, this reason was generally regarded as not important given the relatively low percentage of respondents expressing this sentiment.

The results of the analysis of the likelihood of use of BC methods and products are reported in **Table 10**. Out of the seven independent variables, five were statistically significant in influencing the likelihood of the use of these products. The statistically significant variables included the formal educational attainment of the male respondent and also the educational attainment of his spouse. However, highly educated male respondents who were married to highly-educated female partners had decreased likelihood of using BC methods and products. As expected, the level of awareness of BC methods and products led to increased likelihood of the use of these products.

Explanatory Variable	Regression Parameter Estimate	Student t Value	Probability Level of Significance
INTERCEPT	−16.638	7.832	0.005***
MALEAGE	−0.013	0.183	0.669
MALEEDU	1.210	5.186	0.023**
SPOUSEEDU	0.572	3.778	0.052*
MALEEDU*SPOUSEEDU	−0.052	3.512	0.061*
PINCOMEM	−0.001	0.284	0.594
BCPAWARENES	4.550	7.342	0.007***
BCPAWARENESS*MALEEDU	−0.306	4.331	0.037**

Number of observations for regression analysis was 300 and % observations correct was 86.7. Dependent Variable is log (PROBUSEBCP/1-PROBUSEBCP) (the natural logarithm of the odds ratio in favor of use of BC products and contraceptives).
****Statistical significance of the parameter at the 1% level.**Statistical significance of the parameter at the 5% level.*
**Statistical significance of the parameter at the 10% level.*

Table 10.
Binary logit regression analysis of the current use of birth control products and contraceptives versus selected socio-economic characteristics of the respondents.

Further, when the level of awareness was combined with the educational attainment, the likelihood of the use of BC methods and products declined. This particular result would suggest that male respondents who had relatively lower levels of formal educational attainment were more likely to use BC methods and products when they had increasing levels of awareness information about these products. Hence, this result paved the way for more aggressive forms of publicity of information about BC methods and products targeted at relatively lower educated male respondents.

The results of the regression analysis of the linkage between economic welfare of the male respondents, as indicated by his adjusted personal income, acting as the dependent variable, and various independent variables including the ever-use of BC products are reported in **Table 11**. Using the popular Ramsey Reset test of model specification [28], the model reported in **Table 11** was adequately specified with the Ramsey Reset probability (p) value of rejection of the null hypothesis of correct specification being 0.168 above the critical p value of 0.10 used in the study. Based on the Lagrange Multiplier (LM) test of heteroscedasticity [29], the model also had no significant heteroscedasticity. The power of the model as measured by the R^2 was 0.22; this value would be considered to be modest.

The results shown in **Table 11** indicate that the parameters of all the independent variables were statistically significant. The positive enhancing effects on the economic welfare of the male respondent were due to the status of the person being currently married and also being Muslim. The significant parameters related to the two age variables indicated the existence of a curvilinear relationship between age and economic welfare, consistent with the reproductive life cycle hypothesis used in this study. Differentiating the estimated economic welfare equation with respect to age, the age at which economic welfare started to increase was 47.8 years, assuming other things constant.

The result dealing with the MALEEDUSSS variable showed that respondents who completed secondary school education had significantly lower levels of economic

Variable	Parameter Estimate	Standardized Estimate	T value	Significance probability
	120.977	0.000	6.113	0.000***
MALEAGE	−0.239	−1.627	−2.686	0.008***
MALEAGESQUARED	0.003	1.431	2.397	0.017**
MALEEDUSSS	−2.169	−0.535	−6.237	0.000***
CUMARRIED	0.164	0.097	1.836	0.067*
ISLAMREL	0.987	0.170	3.061	0.002***
HHSIZELARGE	−1.610	−0.427	−6.526	0.000***
EVERUSEDBCP*HHSIZELARGE	0.377	0.167	3.077	0.002***

R^2 = 0.240 Adjusted R^2 = 0.222. Dependent Variable is the natural logarithm of the average monthly personal income of male respondent adjusted for by household size (LPINCOMEM). Significance level of Ramsey Reset test of correct model specification 0.168. Significance level of Lagrange Multiplier (LM) test of heteroscedasticity 0.140.

Table 11.
Regression analysis results of the relationships between a male respondent's economic welfare indicated by his adjusted personal income versus his use of contraceptives and his other socio-economic characteristics.

welfare than other respondents with different types of educational attainments, ranging from no schooling to completion of university education. Increasing household size led to declining economic welfare of the male respondent given the burden of larger household sizes. The effect of the use of BC products and contraceptives in larger-sized households was established. There was positive enhancing effect on the economic welfare of the male respondent from the use of these products for households of sizes, three or more. Thus, households that have started producing children benefitted from the use of these products, possibly due to increased levels of choices to earn incomes, arising from more spacing of births.

5. Conclusions and discussion of policy implication of the study

5.1 Summary of major findings and conclusions

This paper reports the findings of a survey of 300 adult males in all 39 communities of the Amasaman Area Council, Accra, Ghana that elicited information on the perceptions and use of BC products and contraceptives. Nine different BC methods, products and contraceptives were used by the male respondents. Peers and friends were the major source of information about these products. The educational attainment of the male respondent and that of his spouse were statistically significant in increasing the likelihood of use of BC products and contraceptives by the male respondents.

As expected, the degree of awareness of BC products and contraceptives significantly influenced the likelihood of use of these products. Awareness also acted as a moderating variable with combination of formal educational attainment of the male respondent in influencing the likelihood of current use of birth control methods in a negative fashion. This result suggested that males with lower levels of formal educational attainment, and who had higher awareness of BC products and contraceptives, were more likely to use these products.

Economic welfare was shown to be higher for married male respondents than those who were not married. Muslim respondents had significantly higher average income than non-Muslims. The significant parameters related to the two age variables indicated the existence of a curvilinear relationship between the age of the male respondent and his economic welfare; this result was consistent with the reproductive life cycle hypothesis used in this study. Average income of the male respondents increased from 47 years of age onwards.

As expected, larger household sizes were associated with lower levels of economic welfare. However, the ever-use of BC products and contraceptives, in families with larger household sizes, led to increased economic welfare. Given that larger household sizes were defined in the analysis as a dummy variable to denote household sizes of three or more people, this classification would indicate that large households were those involving a married couple with at least one child or dependent. Hence, the economic welfare enhancement obtained from use of BC products and contraceptives was a benefit accruing to households with children.

5.2 New contributions and policy implications arising from the study

This paper makes three contributions to the existing literature dealing with the use of BC products and contraceptives by males and the related policy implications arising from the pattern of male behavior identified in this study. The first contribution is that this study indicated the expected result that increasing awareness of BC products and contraceptives led to the increased likelihood of use of these products by the adult males. Further, it was shown that the increasing awareness of these products for less educated respondents led to increased likelihood of their use by these people. This result would suggest that educational and publicity campaigns of State and Community organizations should target more resources and efforts in RH care and delivery to the less educated sections of the adult male population. The current approach of non-targeted informational programmes, based on uniform spread of awareness messages across the general population of men, may not be very productive.

The second contribution of the study is related to the establishment of evidence of increased economic welfare of male household heads due to the use of BC products and contraceptives, and particularly for those adult males with larger household sizes; this result was possibly due to the increased spacing of births achieved through the use of these products. This result would suggest that targeting of awareness campaigns related to these products would also need to put emphasis on men with large household sizes as they would benefit more in terms of economic welfare arising from the use of these products.

The third contribution of this paper, which closes a gap in the literature, is the finding of very high awareness by the respondents of the traditional Ghanaian method of birth control and family planning related to the male partner avoiding sex with his spouse/partner for a period of time, often one year or more. Despite its very high awareness, and its pre-eminent ranking as the most well-known form of birth control method, among the 300 responding adult males in this study, only about four percent of the respondents were using or had used this method of birth control. This would suggest the need of policy makers and State and community organizations involved with RH care and delivery to bring back the emphasis on the traditional method of birth control related to controlled abstinence after the delivery of children by the spouses and partners of males.

DOI: http://dx.doi.org/10.5772/intechopen.111859

Generally, religious and cultural barriers against the use of birth control methods and products were not considered important by the respondents as they were ranked as reasons for non-use of BC products by less than 10% of the sampled respondents. This result would suggest that the low use of traditional abstinence birth control method was largely related to the information market failure problem; this could be resolved by repeated messaging of its importance by State and Community organizations involved in RH care and delivery to adult males in Ghana.

Acknowledgements

The author thanks all the 300 male respondents for participating in the study. The study was conducted as part of the author's doctoral research work at the Nobel International Business School, Accra, Ghana. The author completed her doctoral research work in December 2021. She received no external funding for this research study. I acknowledge contribution and effort of my research assistant Dennis Nii-Okai Aryee MBA; and the assistance of Professor Kwabena Asomanin Anaman of the Department of Agricultural Economics and Agribusiness, University of Ghana in the development of the statistical models.

Author details

Hanny-Sherry Ayittey
Integrated Investments, Accra, Ghana

*Address all correspondence to: sayite@gmail.com

References

[1] Starbird E, Norton M, Marcus R. Investing in family planning: Key to achieving the sustainable development goals. Global Health: Science and Practice. 2016;**4**(2):191-210

[2] Kriel Y, Milford C, Cordero J, Suleman F, Beksinska M, Steyn P, et al. Male partner influence on family planning and contraceptive use: Perspectives from community members and health care providers in KwaZulu-Natal. South Africa. Reproductive Health. 2019;**16**:89

[3] Gopal P, Fisher D, Seruwagi G, Taddese HB. Male involvement in reproductive, maternal, newborn, and child health: Evaluating gaps between policy and practice in Uganda. Reproductive Health. 2020;**17**(1):114

[4] Basu AM. ICPD: What about men's rights and women's responsibilities? Health Transition Review. 1996;**6**(2): 225-227

[5] Buah FK. A History of Ghana. London: MacMillan; 1998

[6] Ghana Statistical Service (GSS). Annual 2013 to 2022 GDP. Accra: GSS (April); 2023

[7] Ghana Statistical Service (GSS). 2021 National Population and Housing Census: Analytical Report. Accra: GSS; 2021

[8] Anaman KA, Bukari GA. Voter turnouts in presidential elections in Ghana: A political economy analysis using district-level data. Applied Economics and Finance. 2021;**8**(1):13-31. DOI: 11114/aef.v8i1.5083

[9] Abubakari MM, Anaman KA, Ahene-Codjoe AA. Urbanization and arable land use in northern Ghana: A case study of the Sagnarigu municipality in the greater tamale area. Applied Economics and Finance. 2022;**9**(1):68-84

[10] Oxfam International. Ghana: Extreme Inequality in Numbers. London: Oxfam; 2023

[11] Modiglani F. The life cycle hypothesis of saving, the demand for wealth and the supply of capital. Social Research. 1966;**33**(2):160-217

[12] Hindin MJ, Christiansen CS, Ferguson BJ. Setting research priorities for adolescent sexual and reproductive health in low-and middle-income countries. Bulletin of the World Health Organization. 2013;**91**:10-18

[13] Stephenson R, Baschieri A, Clements S, Hennink M, Madise N. Contextual influences on modern contraceptive use in sub-Saharan Africa. American Journal of Public Health. 2007;**97**(7):1233-1240

[14] Nair S, Dixit A, Ghule M, Battala M, Gajanan V, Dasgupta A, et al. Health care providers' perspectives on delivering gender equity focused family planning program for young married couples in a cluster randomized controlled trial in rural Maharashtra. India. Gates Open Research. 2019;**3**:1508

[15] Sedgh G, Ashford LS, Hussain R. Unmet Need for Contraception in Developing Countries: Examining Women's Reasons for Not Using a Method. New York: Guttmacher Institute; 2016

[16] Gizaw A, Regassa N. Family planning services utilization in mojo town, Ethiopia: A population-based study. Journal of Geography and Regional Planning. 2011;**4**(6):355-363

[17] De Silva T, Tenreyro S. Population control policies and fertility convergence. Journal of Economic Perspectives. 2017;**31**(4):205-228

[18] Hawkes S, Hart G. Men's sexual health matters: Promoting reproductive health in an international context. Tropical Medicine and International Health. 2000;**5**(7):A37-A44

[19] Titaley CR, Wijayanti RU, Damayanti R, Setiawan AD, Dachlia D, Siagian F, et al. Increasing the uptake of long-acting and permanent methods of family planning: A qualitative study with village midwives in East Java and Nusa Tenggara Barat provinces, Indonesia. Midwifery. 2017;**53**:55-62

[20] Anaman KA. Research Methods in Economics and Other Social Sciences. Second ed. Saarbrucken, Germany: LAP Lambert Academic Publishing; 2014

[21] Babbie ER. The Practice of Social Research. 15th ed. New York: Cengage; 2020

[22] De Vaus DA. Surveys in Social Research. Sixth ed. London: Routledge; 2014

[23] Gujarati N. Basic Econometrics. Fifth ed. London: McGraw-Hill; 2009

[24] Buse RC, Salathe LE. Adult equivalent scales: an alternative approach. American Journal of Agricultural Economics. 1978;**60**(3): 460-468. DOI: 10.2307/1239943

[25] Anaman KA, Okai JOA. Extent of awareness of birth control methods and their use by women in a peri-urban area of Accra, Ghana. Modern Economy. 2016;**7**:39-54

[26] Apanga PA, Adam MA. Factors influencing the uptake of family planning services in the Talensi District, Ghana. Pan African Medical Journal. 2015;**20**:10. DOI: 10.11604/pamj.2015.20.10.5301

[27] Beson P, Appiah R, Adomah-Afari A. Modern contraceptive use among reproductive-aged women in Ghana: Prevalence, predictors, and policy implications. BMC Women's Health. 2018;**18**(1):157. DOI: 10.1186/s12905-018-0649-2

[28] Ramsey JS. Tests for specification errors in classical linear least squares regression. Journal of the Royal Statistical Society, Series B. 1969;**31**:350-371. DOI: 10.1111/j.2517-6161.1969.tb00796.x

[29] Breusch TS, Pagan AR. A simple test for heteroskedasticity and random coefficient variation. Econometrica. 1979;**47**(5):1287-1294. DOI: 10.2307/1911963

Chapter 10

Family Planning Helps the World

Richard Grossman

Abstract

It is generally recognized that voluntary family planning is essential for the lives and health of individuals in today's world. What is less frequently acknowledged is that family planning has decreased the growth of human population over the past decades. Despite many wonderful advances since the industrial revolution, humans have caused massive deterioration of the natural world. Examples include climate disruption caused by the increase in greenhouse gases and the sixth mass extinction of species. Without modern, voluntary family planning, these negative effects would have been greater. This chapter recommends increased attention to the global public health benefits of family planning by reducing the numbers of unintended births and thus the number of people contributing to our environmental deterioration.

Keywords: contraception, abortion, environment, social justice, public health

1. Introduction

> *Family planning is the most humane vehicle for achieving sustainable social and environmental justice.*
>
> *Jensen and Creinin*

We are accustomed to think of the advantages of Family Planning (FP) to individuals and perhaps to families, but not of the global benefits. This chapter mainly focuses on these benefits to society and to our environment. Throughout the chapter I include access to safe abortion services along with FP [1].

First, I would like to mention the need for more methods of FP, especially for men. At present we have a large variety of methods for women. However, no method is acceptable to all women, and no method is failure-free. Hopefully, improved FP methods will continue to be developed, for both women and men.

In addition, I need to admit to the lack of equity. FP is available to most people in rich countries. However, even in one of the richest countries, the USA, there are geographic locations where it is difficult to access FP services. This has been improved by telemedicine and also by the ability to get FP, including birth control pills, by mail. Nevertheless, there are "abortion deserts", where a woman has to travel long distances in order to abort an unwanted pregnancy. With today's political climate in the USA, access to safe abortion services even is more difficult.

One might think that distance should be no problem in countries with good transportation, however, this is not so. A study performed in the USA has shown that when there is a FP clinic is close to a high school, female students are less likely to drop out of school [2].

IntechOpen

Access to FP services in developing countries is often difficult if not impossible. The difficulty is because of multiple factors including distance, language differences and "stock outs". Often cultural and religious beliefs are serious barriers to accessing and using FP [3].

It is unfortunate that there is no perfect contraceptive method for women, and there is much less available for men. As I write this (April, 2023), I am pleased to note that new oral contraceptive is available that may be safer than past combination pills. Drospirenone/estrol (Nextstellis®) is available in the USA, but is very expensive for those who do not have adequate insurance coverage. Progestin-only oral contraceptives have been around for decades. The have a record of great safety, although breakthrough bleeding and pregnancy rates may be higher than with combined oral contraceptives. Despite the excellent record of safety, the FDA currently requires a prescription for a woman to purchase progestin-only pills. Thanks to the organization "Free the Pill" in the USA our FDA is looking at making this pill available over-the-counter, which will help reduce its cost and make it more accessible.

2. Benefits to the individual

Contraception allows women to enjoy sex with little worry about unintended pregnancy. This permits a woman to finish her education and to start a career before parenting, if that is what she chooses to do. The role of women in developed countries has changed markedly in the 60+ years since oral contraceptives first became available. Although there have been many other factors causing these changes, certainly "the pill" has had a major effect.

Family planning has been called one of the top 10 public health achievements of the 20th century by the US Centers for Disease Control [4]. It allows for longer intervals between the births of children and for smaller family size. By decreasing the number of pregnancies a woman has in her lifetime and increasing intervals between pregnancies, FP has also reduced the mortality and morbidity of women. Because of the longer birth interval, and because each child can receive more resources, FP has helped to save children's lives—especially in developing countries. Improved barrier methods, such as female condoms and nonlatex male condoms, have decreased transmission of HIV and other sexually transmitted infections.

We now have LARCs—Long-Acting Reversible Contraceptives, including hormonal implants and several IUDs. LARCs have very low failure rates, partly because they do not require doing something (such as taking a pill) on a regular basis. Most of the IUDs available in the USA are hormonal. These are being evaluated to find out if they are effective for use longer than their original approval [5]. In addition, they may be useful for postcoital (emergency) contraceptive use [6].

Copper containing IUDs, such as the T 380A (Paragard®), are also very effective for emergency contraception, if inserted within 5 days of unprotected intercourse. Other emergency contraceptive methods include levonorgestrel tablets (which are available without a prescription in many countries) and ulipristal. Although supplanted by more effective methods of emergency contraception, in some areas the only available method may be the Yuzpe regimen. This is using oral contraceptive pills containing ethinyl estradiol and norgestrel, although other formulations may also be effective. Current research has found that emergency contraceptive pills do not work by causing an abortion.

There are many good sources for information about birth control. One that is objective and geared to people in the USA is: www.plannedparenthood.org. The World Health Organization (www.who.int) is a good worldwide source for information.

3. Abortion

There are estimated to be 121 million unintended pregnancies worldwide each year [7]. Some of these are miscarried, some intentionally aborted and some go to term. The World Health Organization states that, globally, about 60% of unintended pregnancies are aborted, and almost half of the abortions are "unsafe". They estimate the total number of global induced abortions at 73 million annually [7].

"Unsafe abortion" is the term that is often used for abortions that are performed outside of the medical system. Usually these abortions are expensive, exploitive and dangerous. Women choose to have an unsafe abortion when they live where abortion is illegal or severely restricted. The risks of an unsafe abortion include serious illness such as hemorrhage or infection, and may result in sterility or death.

It is interesting that abortion is no less common in countries where it is illegal [7]. Perhaps this is because many of these countries also limit access to contraception. Many of the countries where abortion is illegal have high levels of patriarchy and religiosity, with the beliefs that sex should only happen within a marriage. This goes along with limited or no sexuality education, so young women are likely to not be prepared to deal with aggressive males.

4. Global benefits of family planning

The main thrust of this chapter is the benefits of FP to humans, other species and to the environment. I will look at examples in order to make the point that, in addition to helping us, FP helps us to preserve biodiversity and decrease environmental impact.

Most of the world's environmental problems, including climate disruption and loss of biodiversity, would be improved if there were fewer people on the planet. During the past century we have seen remarkable decreases in the rate of population growth, largely due to the use of voluntary FP. Unfortunately, the importance of FP and its relationship to population growth has been largely overlooked by medical and public health people. Furthermore, some people involved in the social sciences seem to actively deny that the planet is overpopulated [8]. Much of this denial comes from religious beliefs and from the regrettable past history of genocide, forced sterilization and eugenics [9].

The good news is that almost half of the world's countries have a total fertility rate (TFR) of less than 2.1, which is the number for replacement fertility [10]. This means that their population will decrease, if the fertility stays below that number, although it may take several decades for that to happen.

How large can the human population be and still be sustainable? I like to use the Ecological Footprint (EF) to compare how we are using Earth's resources with what is available. In short, the EF breaks down our use of resources to land area—land on which to live, to raise food, to develop resources and to dispose of waste.

Globally, there are about 12.2 billion hectares of bioproductive land and of water. Shared evenly among the current roughly 8 billion people on earth, that would be about 1.5 hectares (3.75 acres) for each person. However, many people use more than that. For instance, the average EF for a person in the USA is about 7 hectares (17.2 acres).

The average Ecological Footprint for everyone on Earth is 2.77 hectares—significantly larger than the 1.5 acres that are available. As a consequence, we are using the earth's resources faster than they can regenerate. Calculations suggest that it would take 1.8 planets Earth to support all the humans at the rate at which we are using resources and generating waste. The excess over what the planet can support sustainably is called "overshoot" [11].

One way to calculate a sustainable human population is to divide our current population by the overshoot fraction—8 billion divided by 1.75, or about 4.5 billion people. Unfortunately, one of the shortcomings of the EF is that it does not allow any resources for nonhuman species. With a small allowance for all other flora and fauna, we might find that 4 billion humans would be a sustainable population. If we want the planet to be really healthy, the human population should be about 3 billion people.

There are other, perhaps more accurate ways of calculating the size of a sustainable human population. Mostly they end up with estimates in the range of 2 to 3 billion people, as stated above. For a readable review of this subject, I suggest the book "A Planet of 3 Billion" by Christopher Tucker for more information about a sustainable human population.

The bottom line is that our current human population is not sustainable. In fact, our current population, with the average consumption, is about 2 or 3 times what could be maintained indefinitely. Without modern FP, our numbers would have been much, much larger than the current 8 billion!

Let me explain why I focus on population rather than on consumption. In the formula that describes human impact on the environment, $I = P \times A \times T$ (Impact equals Population times Affluence (or Consumption) times Technology), population is just as important as affluence. However, remember that there are more than 120 million unintended pregnancies every year! [12]. That means that there are many, many women who wish to have control over their fertility—but I know very few people who wish to decrease their affluence. Indeed, globally we live in a sea of advertisements and other media that urge us to buy and consume more, not less.

I do not give the T in the above formula much attention. For instance, I've replaced the lightbulbs in our home with compact fluorescent light bulbs, then with LEDs. We have solar panels on our roof that make most of our electricity and also power our plug-in hybrid vehicle. However, my wife's and my Ecological Footprint is still much larger than 1.5 acres, since these technological modifications only reduce our impact slightly.

To sum up, it would be great to have everyone decrease their footprints down to what is available (1.5 hectares) if we all shared equally. Unfortunately, that is very unlikely. For the average person in the USA it would mean shrinking their footprint by almost 80%, from 7 to 1.5 hectares! Imagine what it would take to have such a small footprint. There are so many things you could not do, and so many things you'd have to do without to have such a small footprint. You would probably have to live in a small house, eat primarily beans and rice or other simple foods with very little meat or none at all. You would have to walk, bike or take public transportation; a car would be impossible. You would have no frills, no TV and probably lots of hard work. It is no wonder that people are not enthusiastic about decreasing their consumption!

On the other hand, millions of people already are trying to control their fertility. Over half a million abortions are performed every year in the USA [13]. It is estimated that there are about 121 million unintended pregnancies globally [7]. The number of women who do not have access to effective contraceptive methods is estimated to be 218 million [14]. Access to voluntary contraception and abortion are certainly the "low hanging fruit" when it comes to decreasing human impact.

There are other, more quantitative ways to appraise the role of FP in lowering our impact [15]. In this part of the discussion, I would like to use climate disruption caused by carbon dioxide (and other greenhouse gasses) as a proxy for all anthropogenic environmental problems. This is because climate disruption is in everyone's mind—as well it should be. Furthermore, climate disruption has been studied a great deal, and in more quantitative ways, than other environmental problem.

For various reasons, the potential for FP to help solve the evolving disaster of climate disruption has been given much less attention than it deserves [16]. An article written in 2010 claims: "Using an energy–economic growth model that accounts for a range of demographic dynamics, we show that slowing population growth could provide 16–29% of the emissions reductions suggested to be necessary by 2050 to avoid dangerous climate change" [17]. Although it may be too late to achieve such a benefit by the year 2050, there are still large advantages to supporting FP for further in the future. Another study suggests that not only is FP effective, but it may be the least expensive means to slow climate disruption [18]. Another article gives an overview of CO_2 emissions in the past and projections using demographics [15].

However, there are other environmental problems than just climate disruption. Extinction of species, global toxification and other impending tragedies may be as bad as, or even worse, than climate disruption. Working together, all this deterioration of the environment will cause problems that we can only begin to imagine. Do not forget that all of these problems are anthropogenic!

5. What could be worse than climate disruption?

Most people understand the CO2 that we emit is caused by people using fossil fuels. However, the connection between human endeavor and the extinction of species may not be so obvious. What is the association between humans and extinction of species? There are a half dozen ways that we are accelerating the loss of species. Paleontologists have known that species have always become extinct, and estimate that the baseline rate is in the range of 1 per million living species per year. The current estimated rate is at least 100 times that, and probably 1000 times or more. One estimate is that there are 8.7 million species on earth and in the oceans [19]. Using the most likely rate of extinction, that would suggest that more than 8000 are being driven to extinction each year. This has been called the "sixth mass extinction" [20].

The biggest reason for extinctions is loss of habitat. Many species of plants and animals require specific conditions to thrive. There are also species, called "endemics", that only live in small areas. If their habitat is disturbed, they die. This is the reason for the Endangered Species Act in the USA. Before any significant development is allowed to occur, the Act requires a survey looking for endangered species. It is sad that all other countries do not have similar laws, and that often the laws (where they exist) aren't always enforced. Unfortunately, the press of the growing human population has already caused the extinction of many species. Joni Mitchel sums it up well in her song, Big Yellow Taxi: "They paved paradise and put up a parking lot [21]".

Each human on the planet requires a place to live and food to eat. The species who had lived on the land before us are evicted; unfortunately, those individuals who survive the bulldozers frequently have no place to go. Often the land used to grow our food is treated with chemicals that are incompatible with the life that had been there [22]. Nonhuman species are being challenged and too often killed off by our civilization in a variety of ways.

Briefly, here are the five other ways that we are causing species to go extinct: (1). The changing climate makes it difficult for some species. For instance, the pika is sensitive to heat. It is a small mammal that lives in cold, mountainous regions. As the climate gets hotter, it can move up in altitude to stay cool. However, they will have no place to go when the mountain tops aren't cold enough. (2). Humans have introduced diseases, such as the fungus that causes white nose syndrome in bats. It is killing susceptible species of bats—which destroy untold numbers of pest insects. (3). We have also introduced exotic species that out-compete vulnerable local species. An example is the salt cedar or tamarisk, which has locally displaced native trees such cottonwoods. (4). In the last century chemists have synthesized thousands of new chemicals. Even though they are given cursory testing for safety before being marketed, some of them have had disastrous unintended consequences. DDT is an example of a chemical with severe unintended consequences [23]. (5). Finally, human greed has killed off some species. Carolina parakeets were numerous at one time, but their colorful plumage became fashionable for ladies' hats. These beautiful birds were hunted to extinction.

We do not know how we will be affected by the mass extinction of other species. We do know that we are a part of the web of life, and that all parts of the web are interdependent. To some extent, all species are important, although some are much more important than others. As our understanding of this web increases, we find out that some species that we thought were of little import are actually essential. Slime molds are an example. They appear unbidden in gardens and woods as unwelcome guests; some of them look like someone vomited on the ground. However, they are helpful because they recycle nutrients [24].

Humans have invested in developing just a few species for our nourishment. Much of our food comes from only a few crops, such as wheat and rice. Likewise, much of the meat we eat comes from just a few species of animals, such as pigs and goats. Although this permits efficient factory farming, it makes us very dependent on just a few species of plants and animals. When there is a disease such as the potato blight in Ireland, this lack of diversity may cause a famine. This is just one way that decreasing biodiversity can affect us. Some experts worry that the mass extinction may be even more problematic to humankind than climate disruption [25].

6. What can we do?

I have several suggestions. Perhaps my strongest recommendation is to support people and organizations that work in the field of reproductive health. This might mean making donations to organizations and clinics that provide FP services. It could mean lobbying politicians who recognize the importance of FP—and it certainly means remembering the importance of FP when it is time to vote.

For those of us in the field of family planning, here is encouragement:

> *"As family planning specialists, we should devote part of our effort to educating policy leaders and the public about the importance of our work from an environmental standpoint" [1].*

Although an individual cannot cure the ills of the world single-handedly, supporting access to family planning is one way that each of us can work to help with climate disruption and also with loss of biodiversity.

Summary

Most of the readers of this chapter are already aware of the advantages of modern family planning—the ability to have sexual intercourse with little fear of an unintended pregnancy. Contraception and abortion have slowed the growth of the human population. Nevertheless, the human numbers are currently 2 or 3 times what would be sustainable. It is important to recognize the important role that family planning plays in helping the non-human portion of the world, in addition to the how it serves people.

Author details

Richard Grossman
Department of Biology, Fort Lewis College, Bayfield, Colorado, USA

*Address all correspondence to: richard@population-matters.org

References

[1] Jensen JT, Creinin MD. Family planning, population growth, and the environment. Contraception. 2020;**101**:145-147. DOI: 10.1016/j.contraception.2020.02.003

[2] Hicks-Courant K, Schwartz AL. Local access to family planning services and female high school dropout rates. Obstetrics and Gynecology. 2016;**127**(4):699-705. DOI: 10.1097/aog.0000000000001344

[3] Adongo PB, Phillips JF, Kajihara B, Fayorsey C, Debpuur C, Binka FN. Cultural factors constraining the introduction of family planning among the Kassena-Nankana of northern Ghana. Social Science & Medicine. 1997;**45**(12):1789-1804. DOI: 10.1016/s0277-9536(97)00110-x

[4] Center for Disease Control and Prevention. Ten great public health achievements--United States, 1900-1999. MMWR. 1999;**48**(12):241-243

[5] Dethier D, Qasba N, Kaneshiro B. Society of Family Planning clinical recommendation: Extended use of long-acting reversible contraception. Contraception. 2022;**113**:13-18. DOI: 10.1016/j.contraception.2022.06.003

[6] Turok DK, Gero A, Simmons RG, Kaiser JE, Stoddard GJ, Sexsmith CD, et al. Levonorgestrel vs. copper intrauterine devices for emergency contraception. New England Journal of Medicine. 2021;**384**:335-344. DOI: 10.1056/NEJMoa2022141

[7] Bearak J et al. Unintended pregnancy and abortion by income, region, and the legal status of abortion: estimates from a comprehensive model for 1990-2019. Lancet Global Health. 2020;**8**(9):E1152-E1161. DOI: 10.1016/S2214-109X(20)30315-6

[8] O'Sullivan, J. The Overpopulation Project. History was rewritten to delegitimize population concerns: we need to reassert the truth. 2022. Available from: https://overpopulation-project.com/history-was-rewritten-to-delegitimize-population-concerns-we-need-to-reassert-the-truth/ [Accessed: April 26, 2023]

[9] Center for Biological Diversity. How to Bring Anti-racism Into the Population Conversation. Available from: https://www.biologicaldiversity.org/programs/population_and_sustainability/population/anti_racism_in_population_conversations.html?utm_source=popx&utm_medium=email&utm_campaign=popx140&emci=6d767997-c60d-ed11-b47a-281878b83d8a&emdi=5de2fa2f-cd0e-ed11-b47a-281878b83d8a&ceid=209594 [Accessed: April 26, 2023]

[10] United Nations Department of Economic and Social Affairs, Population Division. World Population Prospects 2022 (Complete version). Available from: https://population.un.org/wpp/Download/Standard/MostUsed/ [Accessed: April 26, 2023]

[11] Footprint Network. 2023. National Footprint and Biocapacity Accounts. Available from: https://data.footprintnetwork.org/?_ga=2.164379580.263543584.1682351781-264756723.1682351781#/ [Accessed: April 24, 2023]

[12] Ehrlich PR, Holdren JP. Impact of population growth: Complacency concerning this component of man's predicament is unjustified

and counterproductive. Science. 1971;**171**:1212-1217

[13] Centers for Disease Control and Prevention. Abortion Surveillance—Findings and Reports. 2020. Available from: https://www.cdc.gov/reproductivehealth/data_stats/abortion.htm [Accessed: April 24, 2023]

[14] Sully EA, Biddlecom A, Darroch JE, Riley T, Ashford LS, Lince-Deroche N, et al. Adding it up: Investing in Sexual and Reproductive Health. New York: Guttmacher Institute 2019. 2020. Available from: https://www.guttmacher.org/report/adding-it-up-investing-in-sexual-reproductive-health-2019 [Accessed: April 24, 2023]

[15] O'Neill BC, Liddle B, Jiang L, Smith KR, Pachauri S, Dalton M, et al. Demographic change and carbon dioxide emissions. Lancet. 2012;**380**:157-164. DOI: 10.1016/S0140-6736(12)60958-1

[16] Bongaarts J, O'Neill BC. Global warming policy: Is population left out in the cold? Population policies offer options to lessen climate risks Science. 2018;**361**(6403):650-652. DOI: 10.1126/science.aat8680

[17] O'Neill BC, Dalton M, Fuchs R, Jiang L, Pachauric S, Zigovad K. Global demographic trends and future carbon emissions. PNAS. 2010;**107**(41):17521-17526

[18] Yan Feng et al. Data Analysis of Reducing CO2 Emissions by Investing in Family Planning. 2015. Available from: https://populationmatters.org/resources/data-analysis-of-reducing-co2-emissions-by-investing-in-family-planning/ [Accessed: April 26, 2023]

[19] Mora C, Tittensor DP, Adl S, Simpson AGB, Worm B. How many species are there on earth and in the ocean? PLoS Biology. 2011;**9**(8):e1001127. DOI: 10.1371/journal.pbio.1001127

[20] Ceballos G, Ehrlich PR, Barnosky AD, García A, Pringle RM, Palmer TM. Accelerated modern human–induced species losses: Entering the sixth mass extinction. Science Advances. 2015;**1**(5):e1400253. DOI: 10.1126/sciadv.1400253

[21] Mitchell J. Big Yellow Taxi. New York: City Siquomb Publishing Corp; 1970

[22] Sodhi NS, Ehrlich PR. Conservation Biology for all. Oxford: Oxford University Press; 2010

[23] Carson R. Silent Spring. Cambridge: Riverside Press; 1962

[24] Helena H. Lichens, Slime Moulds and Wasps: RHS Lists Top Beneficial Wildlife for Garden. The Guardian; 2023. Available from: https://www.theguardian.com/environment/2023/apr/22/lichens-slime-moulds-and-wasps-rhs-lists-top-beneficial-wildlife-for-garden [Accessed: April 24, 2023]

[25] University of Copenhagen. Biodiversity Crisis Is Worse than Climate Change, Experts Say. Science Daily; 2012. Available from: https://www.sciencedaily.com/releases/2012/01/120120010357.htm#:~:text=Biodiversity%20is%20declining%20rapidly%20throughout,global%20climate%20change%2C%20experts%20say.&text=Biodiversity%20is%20declining%20rapidly%20throughout%20the%20world.,-The%20challenges%20of. [Accessed: April 24, 2023]

Chapter 11

Government Sponsored Community-Based Health Extension Program Enhancing Contraceptive Provision in Southern Ethiopia: An Interpretive Phenomenological Exploration

Abraham Alano and Lori Hanson

Abstract

Albeit the government efforts improving access to contraception through health extension programs in Ethiopia, gaps exhibited on experiences of the stakeholder about the basis on services provision. Therefore, perceptions about the enablers and rationale for contraceptive service were explored. Interpretative phenomenological design was employed to explore the lived experiences of stakeholders. Focus group discussions, individual in-depth interviews, and key informant interviews were employed for data collection. Data were analyzed using interpretive phenomenological analysis. The finding indicated that contraceptive service provision from the socio-economic perspectives was understood adequately, but the human rights-based rationale was shadowed. The contribution of the health extension program for contraceptive use has been remarkable. The improvement is attributed to the alignment of primary health care with the community organizations such as women development armies. The health extension program accelerated contraceptive service and given momentum for PHC. Women revealed encouraging involvement in the process of contraceptive service access and use. However, the bigger picture, and rationale for providing contraceptive services, the human rights approach, remained elusive at lower hierarchy. Hence, the study recommends that the disconnect in the broader premises of providing contraceptive services must be properly communicated across the stakeholders.

Keywords: health extension program, human rights, contraception, phenomenology, rationale

1. Introduction

The provision of modern contraceptive services in developing nations began because of the strong push from developed nations in the 1960s [1–4]. However, the lack of strong governments commitments along with limited resources and the underlying socio-cultural factors remain major impediments to the expansion of the services in many developing nations [5]. Among the notable challenges to be mentioned in the process of service provision is the access to contraceptive services affected by a lack of well-structured institutions in terms of the availability of health professionals and material inputs [6].

To narrow the gap between developed and developing nations toward contraceptive service access and use, the Primary Health Care Declaration (PHC) provides guidance that played a significant role [7, 8]. PHC has clarified a meaningful health strategy for reducing maternal and child morbidities and mortalities in developing nations [9]. Moreover, PHC has bridged the gap between institutional health service delivery and community demands through a community-based service delivery modality [10].

Ethiopia has realized that health issues require the involvement of multiple sectors and collective undertakings. Based on this understanding, the country revitalized the primary healthcare approach by identifying key stakeholders and sectors to involve in the implementation of health-related activities and actions [11, 12]. Guided by the health policy of the transitional government, the Federal Ministry of Health of Ethiopia (FMOH) has taken numerous measures to improve the health status of its population. Among the major steps that have been taken in designing and development of A 24 Health Sector Development Plan (HSDP) with its five successive five-year phases is among the several steps the government actions. After a critical evaluation of the health-based initiatives, the MOH revised its approach and incorporated government-paid community-based health service delivery, the health extension program (HEP) in 2003 [13–15].

The HEP is an innovative approach constituting a paradigm shift in Ethiopia's health service delivery creating strong links between the mainstream institutional health service and community-based health service expansion [16]. The peculiar aspect of the health extension program is that the service providers are all women except in a few pastoral villages and permanent employees of the government. They serve in the rural villages where they grew up, live and, are permanent employees of the government. This was different from the former practice which was based on volunteerism.

The HEP is expected to improve access to health care through increased availability and acceptance as workers largely share similar cultural backgrounds and speak the same language as the community they serve [17–19].

In spite of half a century or more contraceptive services in Ethiopia and encouraging engagements of the government and health workers, there are limited research outputs that reveal the depth of the lived experiences of service users, health workers, and health leaders about how service organizations and extension affect the outcome. This study sought to explore the ways that leaders in the health system, health care providers, and service users attempt to create an enabling environment for contraceptive service provision and its use. The study was conducted by aiming to describe patterns of a provision of contraceptive services and capture the perspectives of health care providers, leaders, and service users' and their lived experiences on enabling conditions of the contraceptive service organization, provision, and use.

2. Materials and methods

2.1 The research context

This study was conducted in three districts of Sidama Zone designated by Hawassa University as technology villages for research and technology transfer. The three districts were selected for accessibility. Hawassa University is located in the Sidama Zone, one of the 13 zones in the Southern Nations Nationalities and People's Regional state (SNNPRG) of Ethiopia. Sidama Zone is located in the south-eastern part of the region and is bordered by Oromia Regional state on the south, east and north and with Wolaita Zone in the west [20]. Projected from the 2007 national population census, the zone has a total of 3,471,568 people of which 1,753,142 (50.5%) are men and 1,718,426 (49.5%) are women. Close to 24% of the total population of the zone are estimated to be women of reproductive age. Household family size is estimated to be 4.7 and the annual population growth of the zone is estimated to increase 2.9% [21].

2.2 Study design

The study employed an interpretive (hermeneutic) phenomenological approach which is appropriate for understanding the life world of contraceptive service users women, health care workers (health professionals), and health leaders. It focuses on describing the meanings given by the individuals and how these meanings (the experiences of health care workers, health leaders, and service user women enable contraceptive services provision and use) influence the access to the service and use [22, 23]. The approach further considers the importance of the expert knowledge of the researcher as a valuable guide to the inquiry. The study aims to explore the life experiences related to the enabling conditions for contraceptive services and use by employing this approach. It offered a unique opportunity to establish a rich and in-depth understanding of sustainable and progressive contraceptive services establishment [24].

2.3 Data collection

To capture in-depth information about the topic of interest: focus group discussions (FGDs), individual in-depth interviews, and key informant interviews were used. Three female research assistants with educational and professional experience were employed to fit the majority of study participants (the rural women). Recruiting the research assistants helped to bridge the gap in both language and gender. Recruitment of research assistants was done in consultation with the Regional Health Bureau, Zonal Health Department and colleagues. After recruitment and training the research assistants, health extension workers, and local women, the community leaders collaborated in the selection of study participants. A purposive sampling method was used to include well-informed participants in the study as key informants, focus group discussants, and in-depth interviewees to explore the depth of their lived experiences [25, 26].

Participants were enrolled in the study based on criteria set to suit the study requirement. These include: the women's experiences of the contraceptive services use for at least a year, their ability to elaborate on the services and factors affecting the service access in their locality, and health leaders at different hierarchies (health institute, district, zonal, regional, and ministerial level) and the health extension workers.

A total of 82 women of reproductive age group were included and participated in the focus group discussions comprised of 7–12 participants in each FGD. For the individual in-depth interview, 19 women of reproductive age from nine kebeles were involved. A total of 18 key informants were involved in the interview based on the designated position they hold in their respective institutions (Appendix A). Semi-structured FGDs and interview guides were developed for the interview and the participants were encouraged to speak up about their experiences. This type of interview guide is assumed to be in line with the interpretive phenomenological approach that gives reasonable freedom for the participants to express their experiences of the phenomenon of interest in their ways. It further deepened discussions and reflections on the life experiences of the study participants [27, 28].

Discussions were arranged in consideration of the time and regularity and viability of rural women. All the discussions were conducted outside of market days and from 10:00 A.M. to 11:30 A.M. Data collection schedule was arranged with the study participants through the community health workers (the health extension workers and women development army leader). Consideration was given by the study team on time management as such arriving at the data collection site in time and arranging the setup in a convenient way. The seating arrangement was organized circularly so that everybody could have ample opportunity to properly see one another.

Once the study discussants took their seats, the health extension worker carried out greetings and introduced the research team. Informed consent was obtained to audio-tape and take notes during the discussion. Moderation of the discussion was done primarily by the principal investigator. The research assistant aided by translating to the women and back to the PI and taking the note. A discussion was conducted by giving adequate time that was apportioned for the women to raise issues related to the guiding questions. Care was taken to involve all participants equally so each could discuss their lived experiences. The discussion was managed by considering the standard time for the qualitative data collection and women's busy schedules. Each session lasted 60–90 minutes on average. Discussion sessions concluded with due care about the completeness of the collected data, if there were any queries from the participants and acknowledging their commitment. Participants were informed about the need to attend a subsequent meeting following the preliminary analysis of the first discussion.

The discussion session was recorded using two digital recorders to ensure accuracy and prevent equipment failure. A unique identifier was given to each focus group discussion to differentiate it from subsequent discussions and avoid confusion during transcription. Written notes were taken by a research assistant simultaneously.

Following the focus group discussion, the individual in-depth interviews were conducted with women participants by the research team in the woman's home or at the health post based on the preferences of the interviewee. For those who were interviewed at their home, the research team was guided by the health extension worker or the community leader. A signed consent was obtained from the participants by reading the form out loud to continue the interview. The study team managed the session by providing an even chance to all participants and encouraging all to talk about their life experience in detail without any fear or reservations. In such ways, the interview continued for 40 to 60 minutes until the study team agreed on the emerging ideas as repetitions [29]. Handwritten notes were taken and an audio-tape of the interview was recorded.

Lastly, key informant interviews were conducted in the following manner. Flexible interview dates were arranged as almost all the key informants were busy with their official routines. Once the key informants were identified, an interview schedule was arranged with each interviewer either calling via phone or visiting the office in person. The key informants' interviews were arranged in the informant's office or working unit at a convenient time. The study team managed the interview reaching the site in time to ensure the functionality of materials and give adequate time for the key informants to read the consent form and sign it.

Key informant interviews began by briefly explaining the purpose of the study, the procedures for selecting the informants, and the overall process of the study. Once the research team obtained a final signed consent form from the participant, the interview was conducted. The convenience of the room and the sitting arrangement for the interview was ensured before directly embarking into the interview. By using a semi-structured interview guide, the interview was conducted flexibly and systematically.

The interview process was done by following a qualitative study data collection approach suiting this specific (interpretive phenomenology) design. The interview session was conducted as guided by the study guide questions and opportunities to probe more issues as they emerged. Adequate time was given to capture the necessary information and to ensure the documentation of both handwritten notes and recording the audio-tape. Finally, the research team thanked the informants for their time and information before departing and told them about the possibility of returning for further discussion after the preliminary analysis. All key informant interviews were conducted in similar procedures. Data collection was conducted from September 2013 to May 2014.

2.4 Data analysis

This study used the guiding principles of interpretive phenomenological methodology. It enables viewing the phenomenon along the way that reflects the significant interaction of both the data sources (participants) and the researchers as part of their "being in the world" rather than only "being' itself [30, 31]. Thus, the interinfluence and connections of the two sources are reflected in the interpretive analysis. An adapted flow diagram from the interpretive phenomenological analysis (IPA) was used to guide the analysis (Appendix B).

Data analysis was conducted in two languages. The following steps describe the process: transcriptions were carried out on all the audio-taped materials verbatim, first in Amharic and then in English (Appendix C). Materials were also translated back to Amharic by a professional linguist. After that, the Amharic translation was given to the principal investigator to check for consistency.

Summary finding in the form of shortened transcripts incorporating the field notes was presented to the key informants for their further input and comments. Data immersion by the researcher immersed into the data several times through repeated reading to find out emerging codes. The analysis process utilized several rounds of indulging in the transcripts, reading and rereading, consultation with the key informants, and soliciting their inputs for the emerging descriptive codes. Inputs from the informants were incorporated into the second round of data analysis with remarks. Side notes and descriptive coding were then completed for all the materials. Data reduction was done in a step-by-step approach, beginning with the transcripts, followed by descriptive coding, and then distilling this material into themes by bringing similar ideas and concepts together.

The overall analysis process made use of the hermeneutic circle, which means iterative back-and-forth linkage of data from both the researcher's and participants' perspectives. Guided by the study questions, the side notes, linked to the descriptive codes, themes were identified These steps were done by re-visiting the transcripts after major themes had been identified to interpret connections between the initial data and our later refinements [29, 30, 32]. Summarized reports were presented to study participants about the phenomena derived from their shared experiences. Discussions were held with participants based on the study guide questions and core concepts. Their feedback was incorporated in line with the experience of the researcher. This increased the confidence in interpretations and further enriched the understanding of the phenomena.

Data quality was assured using the steps of qualitative data quality assurance approaches generally called trustworthiness. The four closely resembling criteria for ensuring trustworthiness are credibility (truth value), transferability (applicability), dependability (consistency), and conformability (neutrality) suggested in the literature [33]. Actions carried out to ensure the trustworthiness were: (1) presenting the summary of transcripts to the study participants to give them an opportunity for further comment; (2) reviewing of the preliminary findings to ensure the early findings reflect what they know and experience; (3) sharing the preliminary summary findings with the health managers and service providers to check interpretations.

3. Results

The findings of this study are organized under the respective questions relating to health provider efforts in creating an environment conducive to contraceptive uptake and use. The aim was a better understanding of the issues of service delivery organization, processes, and content related to service availability, accessibility, convenience, trends, and the current status of contraceptive services. Moreover, the pattern of service integration, linkage among the primary health care units and the community organizations, and anticipated challenges related to services sustainability and ensuring quality were also explicated.

3.1 Trends and patterns of contraceptive service provision in connection to the HEP

3.1.1 Health managers and service providers' perspectives

Despite more than half a decade of longevity of the contraceptive service provision in Ethiopia and the study area, the progress in reaching all segments of the population was sluggish. Voluntary non-governmental organizations mainly, the Family Guidance Association of Ethiopia, started this service provision at an early age. Integration of the contraceptive services into health systems took place gradually but service expansion and increment in method mix remained low until 2005, where sharp increment took place since then. All study participants in three data collection methods expressed frankly that the current level of contraceptive services expansion and improvement in the availability of method mix was attributed to the health extension program.

As pointed out by study participants that the health extension program has brought contraceptive services closer to residents living and working places. In doing so, it has improved unconditional access to the service.

The extraordinary contribution of the health extension program in enhancing the contraceptive service access unlike the previous approach, is its propensity to extend the services to the household level through home visits and other community-based distribution options using community-based organizations such as women development armies. Another merit of the health extension workers is that they are female and recruited from the same *kebeles* where they offer service. This created a conducive environment for service-seeker women to feel comfortable when visiting the health post to access contraceptive service and when the female HEW visits their home; they express their needs without reservation. Moreover, the service-providing health extension workers share a similar culture and speak the same language and being female creates a favorable environment for women to ask whatever questions they desire. Study participants substantiated these conclusions:

> *The health extension program has improved access and utilization to communities and households. Gender parity of the health extension workers with plenty of health service users, the women is another important issue received attention. The program played incredible role that averted several barriers of contraceptive service use. These were evidenced by the convenience the program created for women in terms of time, distance language and cultural harmony. On top of the above, the program also created gender parity between the service providers and users. In the nutshell, the health extension program improved access to the services*

> *The health extension program is therefore a reason for the rapid increment in contraceptive prevalence and service coverage in the district as of the last seven years. This is so because the health extension workers provide the service both institutional and outreach models (at health posts but also house to house visitation). The health extension program significantly reduced the former distance of more than 5–10 KM to 2–3 KM walk and stretched it to the household level.*

The finding of the study has justified that the establishment of the health extension program created a strong services link within the primary health care units and the community. This further contributed to the current state of contraceptive use progress. More specifically, community mobilization using women development armies, and a one-to-five network [1] through model households are notable experiences to learn from.

All the study participants consensually remarked that the health extension program and the service organization have functional linkages manifested through collaborative undertakings at the community level. The strong collaborative undertakings between the health extension workers, the women development armies, and a one-to-five community network ensured the expansion of contraceptive service within their catchment area. Such interlinks or collaboration among stakeholders not only improves access to services but also is a clear indication for female empowerment as the service providers, advocators, and community leaders lead contraceptive service programs. This was further substantiated by citations from the study participants and a district-level manager explained the issue as follows:

> *Health system organization in the study area is a witness for the observed strong linkage and collaborative undertakings. The health professionals from the health center provide supportive supervision to the health post and in a similar passion the health extension worker do so for the women development army. The supportive supervision is for all the health extension packages including the family planning services.*

Similarly, another experienced health extension worker has given her experience in this regard by clearly indicating:

> *By its very nature the health extension program is from the 'community to the community', that has strong linkage between the service providers, users and leaders. The relationship is eventually took a shape of strong family and created mutual trust. We, the health extension worker provide service with a sense of serving our fellow women. A woman being the first contact point in the household has been another ease condition for the expansion of services both in the household and the community. On top of the women development army a one-to-five network system, we also use other community organizations such as 'edir' and 'kuteba mehiber [2]'. We work collaboratively with all these organizations, networks and systems. Generally, we have established a strong working relationship starting from an individual woman to the community level.*

3.1.2 Service user women's perspectives

Experiences of service user women toward contraceptive service availability and accessibility in the era of health extension programs are congruent with the health service manager and service providers' articulations.

Women explained that, unlike the previous high-level health institutions, now they comfortably express their feelings and get services including advice easily through understanding. They never fear or feel ashamed of telling their feelings as the health extension workers are from the same localities. When the health extension workers visit clients' houses, women easily talk to them and even invite them to have coffee or food. Because of such interaction, the extension workers feel at home and well-acquainted with the service users. This was not the case before the inception of the health extension program.

Daname, a woman in the focus group discussion who has used contraceptive services from various sources elaborated on the service access difference and the convenience now and previously:

> *I paid 270 ETB for contraceptive service (surgical implant) at Yirgalem hospital before the access to contraceptive service improved. I also waited for five days to get service in addition to paying a service charge as stated above. Now the situation is different. Service accessibility was greatly improved. As the former discussants mentioned, we got service here at our kebele by our children. This is a big change. We share our feelings without hiding anything from the health extension workers. We don't have a problem with waiting for long hours for services, no need to go daily to queue up for services, no one tells us to bring your card from the card room. We receive services at one stop shot.*

Similarly, another woman in one of the focus group discussions vented:

> *More specifically, the establishment of a health post in our kebele has created a better chance to access health services both for ourselves and our children. We were troubled*

> *to access the health services for our children before the establishment of this health post. It was customary to move here and there looking for health services previously. We were forced to take them to medically unproven services and exposed them to unsanitary/unhygienic services. Past years were known for us for the huge deaths of our young children others remained disabled. Appreciation should be paid to the government and our God who brought this time. We got relief and our children are growing well and healthy (Baliessie, a mother of 5 children and 30 years old).*

Loetie, a 25-year-old woman who used contraceptive service for 5 years explained her lived experience as how she has benefited from the service as:

> *Remarkable change is seen here when compared to the earlier time. Instead of waking far distance to access contraceptive service, this time I am accessing contraceptive service here in my kebele with a short walk distance. Before the health extension program, one was experienced walking long distances and required to pay for contraceptive service. Thus, the long-distance walk, time and financial barriers hampered from service users in the pre-health extension era. Grace be to the Almighty God and appreciation to the government; we receive health information daily. The health extension workers provide services and information in all the packages, with due focus on how to keep our hygiene, different types of contraceptive methods available in the health posts and elsewhere, inform the benefits of contraceptive use about spacing pregnancies thereby improving the health status of both mothers and children.*

Furthermore, women expressed their views on the contribution of the health extension workers in creating health services demand and access in their respective kebele. They are the first to bring contraceptive information and services; by the way, this remains the reason for the improved prevalence of service use in their kebele. Women further witnessed that their know-how and skills for health service use are improved since the establishment of the health extension program.

This is further supported by the excerpts from other participants:

> *Before the health extension program, I knew nothing about what contraceptive service mean and why it exists. We hardly find health services in our locality until the establishment of the health post in our kebele. Mostly we were ignorant about health services such as contraceptive use and vaccination. Immediately following the establishment of the health post in our kebele, the worker started to inform us about various health extension packages including contraceptive use and related benefits. They showed us the difference between unplanned and planned fertility and mechanisms to control fertility, (Dalbe, a 27 years old used contraceptives for 7 years).*

A one-to-five network means a model woman in one of the five neighboring households: act as a team leader (due to her outstanding performance on the health extension program) for all development-related affairs in that team.

4. Discussion

4.1 Toward an enabling environment for contraceptive use

The perception of participants in the study regarding the environment in relation to contraceptive service is discussed in this section and includes: (1) the service organization that includes accessibility, availability, acceptability, and convenience (2) the premises of rights approach for service provision and (3) special contributions of health extension program as an innovative primary health care strategy toward contraceptive service.

4.2 Contraceptive service organizations (content and process)

The study has indicated that until recently, the access and availability of services were weak in the country. The findings confirmed this claim, as, at the early stages of the health extension program, only oral contraceptive pills were available at health posts. Currently, couples of methods are available including short-term methods and long-term methods at the health posts provided through a health extension program. However, the availability of more methods is not uniform across the health institution. It increases when one goes up in the hierarchy of health services delivery institutions.

Agreement is established among stakeholders (services providers, users, and health managers) of the availability, accessibility, convenience, and use of contraceptive services in the study area. One can conclude that there are some improvements in coordination and communication among stakeholders concerning the service processes and contents. Except for a few, all the participants' experiences showed that contraceptive service availability, accessibility, and quality are improving. Some peculiarities were experienced concerning the injectable contraceptive method availability of specifically injectable contraceptives.

The lack of a particular method, an injectable contraceptive (which is more likely accepted by users), may pose a challenge to further expanding and sustaining contraceptive services [34]. Switching from one method to another ought to be due to defined medical reasons or the choice of the client, but the current shortage-related switching is another hindrance that may overshadow service quality and expansion. The shortage of widely acceptable contraceptive methods could hamper service expansion and negatively affect the good feedback toward the HEP. The irregularity in availing of preferred methods may contrast with the established service norms, which state that the service delivery should provide adequate attention to socio-cultural and personal experiences [35–37].

The study examined the processes that support the provision of high-quality contraceptive services and revealed that most contraceptive users' access services from health posts. As indicated, the prime source of contraceptive services in the community is the health extension worker with close supervision from the health center. Therefore, maintaining the quality of such service is dependent on regular updating of the competence of the health extension workers through continuous refresher training and supportive supervision. These must be coupled with the provision of materials that help with spot references such as job aid, guidelines, manuals, and standard operating procedures. The availability and use of reference materials are examined in this study from the perspectives of service providers and managers.

The higher-level health service managers argue that they have prepared and distributed standard supportive documents in the form of manuals, flipcharts, and leaflets as requested by the regions. Similarly, most of the health extension workers indicated the availability of reference materials adequately and useful in guiding their service provisions. However, few of the service providers had shared their feelings that the materials are inadequate or incomplete for fulfilling the level of competency required for service provision. The study revealed that reference materials (and that the materials are comprehensive and easy to understand and use) by the service providers helped to provide contraceptive services efficiently. Service providers' competency is crucial for initial service start-up and subsequent continuation of service provision. The findings from USAID-Deliver [38], argue that proper method choice and sustained use are dependent on the information clients receive from providers.

Government-sponsored health extension program is one of the significant indicators for the established links to the contraceptive uptake. The establishment of the health extension program remained a unique landmark for the rapid services uptake and quality improvement. This is further evidenced that more than half a decade-long service remained sluggish in its progress but has shown tremendous improvement since the establishment of this program. As has been indicated in much empirical evidence [39, 40], the service coverage showed tremendous improvement in contraceptive prevalence.

From the perspectives of the service providers, health services managers and users, the study scrutinized their view of which factors contributed to the remarkable improvement in contraceptive use and any defined connection to the new innovative community-based health extension program. Their lived experiences indicated that the health extension program has made a unique contribution to rapidly improving access to and convenience of these services for women. As indicated in the participants' experiences the health extension program improved services access by bringing them closer to women where they live, and work compared with the former strictly institutionalized approach of service delivery.

The availability of the services in each *community organizations* created the opportunity for women to easily access the services tackling challenges related to distance and requirements of permission from their husbands. In circumstances when women maintain the secrecy of their service use from their husbands, they go to the health post as if they are going to a neighbor's house. Studies support this finding that any service to be promoted and used by the target group should fulfill certain conditions including physical, financial, and socio-cultural aspects. Bringing services closer to the potential users increases the possibility of actual use [41, 42].

Another peculiarity of the health extension program concerning contraceptive service is that the program has removed many obstacles and barriers that hampered women's potential for service use. When the behavior of health professionals welcomes the service users (cultural and linguistic congruence) clients are more likely to use services [43, 44]. Thus, this study finding is in congruence with the above one as the health extension workers are almost all women recruited from the *community* which they serve and share the same culture and language. This has removed the gender, language, and cultural barriers between service providers and service users.

The contextual similarity between the health extension workers and service user women not only created a unique opportunity for the early services adoption but also for the continuous use. Women evidently expressed their experiences in this regard by comparing their pre-health extension program service inquiries. Formerly, the service was far from their residential area and male-dominated. Moreover, they were requested to pay for services and in most cases looked for a translator to explain their feelings to the health professional. As a result, they were highly discouraged from the health institutions to seek services [17–19].

The peculiarity of health extension programs in improving access is their conformity to the local community context. The contraceptive service extension to the household through home visits by female health extension workers is favorably welcomed by the community. Program. This is connected to cultural aspects and the domestic work patterns in which most rural women stay home doing domestic duties, and thus, are easily accessible for a health extension worker to provide services during their home visits.

The study further showed another crucial perspective of the health extension program the participants' life worlds related to contraceptive service, its alignment to the multidimensional aspects of the health systems from the health principles and philosophical ascertainments. The organizational arrangement of the health extension program shows strong links from the community level to the mainstream health institution. This further indicated and assured the need for close collaboration across the wide dimensions of actors to ensure the success of the program. The health system closely works with partners at various levels to fill gaps either technically or materially. Many study findings show that health service delivery approaches that do not leave room for inter-sectorial cooperation and that do not ensure community involvement is never satisfactorily accessible, acceptable, or sustainable [19, 39, 43, 44].

More so is the trust the health extension program builds at the community level. It is at this time that the health system closely functions with the local community in a sustainable manner. This is in line with the assertion that the health system is being affected and affects other systems. This is evidenced by that the health extension program functions in a network at the *kebele* level. The health extension workers participate in the *kebele* affairs and receive support from the *kebele* administration. They are members of the *kebele* command post, which is responsible for overall affairs. Furthermore, the health extension workers closely function with the women development armies, one-to-five networks, and model household women. This has established strong linkages between the health extension program and the community members at a basic level. Thus, it is through such channels that information and services flow until they reach the households and target women.

The trust and strong collaboration established between the health extension workers and the current women users of contraception has created a circular passion for the information dissemination to the current non-user women in the community. The platform of current service-user women in the community through the women development army and the one-to-five network in their neighborhood helped initiation of discussion about contraceptive use and its benefits with the current non-user counterparts by sharing their life experiences. Perry and Roger (2014) argue that if the health service delivery approach offers attention to the multiple dimensions of health determinants and involves all stakeholders, the service uptake increases tremendously. Gulzar and Ali [45] also agree that the client's family planning service use behavior is largely influenced by the relationship between the service provider and the client. This study has proved that female health extension workers have greatly improved contraceptive service uptake by extending service to households through home visitation.

The basic premise of contraceptive service provision was reemphasized that the health extension program packages were designed based on fundamental human and reproductive rights. The human rights dimension for reproductive health received little attention at its earliest time. Through the persistent struggle of the advocacy groups coupled with a series of UN conferences, meetings, and treaties have produced an agreed-upon approach to ensure the reproductive health rights of service users. The essence that human beings have a right to enjoy the highest level of attainable health, including sexual and reproductive health, received increased attention. Women and men have the right to have means to do so without any discrimination and coercion. Such ascertainments ensure that women have the right to choose a method best suited to their condition and to withdraw from the method when it fails to do so. In the contrary to the human rights principle, failure to provide adequate information and limiting service access is an indication that the contraceptive service is not in line with the ICPD plan of action. Hardee et al. [46] argue that any family planning program must respect the ICPD plan of action and must guarantee freedom of contraceptive choice and respect, protect, and fulfill human rights.

4.3 Strengths and limitations

The study was conducted in three districts of the Sidama zone and considered only the married women currently using the services may be considered as the limitations of the. Sexual and reproductive matters are usually sensitive and considered as taboo in most rural communities, thus might have limited the depth of response during data collection. Another possible limitation is that the study has not considered current non-users' perceptions of the benefits of contraception. Men are also not considered in this study as the prime purpose of the study is to explore the experiences of women.

The study was carried out to explore the experiences of women contraceptive service users in the Hawassa University research villages, which were established to observe the impact of university-based research in knowledge generation, technology transfer, and the livelihood of the residents. The scope and patterns of this study have taken such shape with the assumption to strengthen the university-community linkage. These are some of the delimitations of this study.

4.4 Conclusion and recommendation

Based on the findings of this study, it can be concluded that the contraceptive service organizations' process and content, are encouraging and improvements made in service quantity and quality. HEP symbolized the effectiveness of community-based health services provision as the backbone of primary health care. Moreover, HEP amicably expressed the functionality of intersectoral collaboration and various community-based organizations networks hand-in-hand for the betterment of the most needy segment of the society. Women revealed encouraging involvement in the process of contraceptive service access and use in their organizations such as development armies and the one-to-five network.

4.5 Recommendations

Identifying successful strategies for the sustainable use of reproductive health services from the human and women's rights perspectives is vital not only to ensure the well-being of women and their significant others but also toward ensuring the attainment of sustainable development goals. This study, therefore, has come up with the following recommendations to ensure evidence-based service provision and propel contraceptive service use in a way that consistently respects human rights and sustainable use:

1. Strengthen the existing community networks through proper evaluation and feedback and create strategies on how to improve men's involvement in reproductive health services, including contraception, in a manner that respects, protects, and fulfills women's rights.

2. Establish mechanisms to share the experiences of women development armies, a one-to-five network to expand the inclusion of men and elders to broaden contraceptive services to the current non-user and ensure sustainability

3. Special preparation is needed to avail of the contraceptive methods without discontinuation

5. Declaration

5.1 Ethical considerations

Ethical clearance for this study was obtained from all concerned institutions both abroad and in-land. These are: the University of Saskatchewan, Canada, Hawassa, University, Ethiopia and the SNNPR Health Bureau, Ethiopia. Study participants offered their consent in written form ensuring their voluntariness to be part of the study. The study team explained the purpose of the study; its benefits and any risk in case thoroughly to prove the confidence of the study participant. Study participants were informed about communication of the study finding in various meetings, workshops and publications and verbal consents were obtained.

5.2 Consent for the publication

This manuscript is an extract from the PhD dissertation with some addition later on. All ethical issues including communication of the finding to various stakeholders were properly communicated and their consents were obtained. Study participants signed consent forms in the local language are attached under the supporting document Section 7.

5.3 Declaration of funding

The original PhD dissertation was funded by the joint contribution of Hawassa University, Ethiopia and the University of Saskatchewan, Canada. The funding was only covered fieldwork expenses such as travel cost, perdiem, fuel, and related incidentals. Additional data were gathered at the expense of the authors' personal pockets. No fund was allocated for the communication of finding such as publication. There is no interference of the funding entities in all undertakings of the study work except offering the fund for the accomplishment of the study.

Authors' contribution

The manuscript is a joint effort of all the authors. AA was responsible for conducting data collection, analysis, and the write up. LH was responsible for revising transcription, analysis, editing, and supervising all steps. MM was involved in designing the study, manuscript preparation, editing of the manuscript.

DOI: http://dx.doi.org/10.5772/intechopen.111694

Competing interest

The manuscript is the efforts of both authors primarily dedicated to academic purposes. The financial support from Hawassa and Saskatchewan universities was in support of a PhD study. The manuscript is partially taken from the PhD dissertation with some addition of data after it. Hence, there were no competing interests either from the funding sources or the authors.

List of abbreviation

WHO	World Health Organization
PHC	Primary Health Care
MOH	Ministry of Health
HEP	Health Extension Program
HEW	Health Extension Worker
SNNPRG	South Nation, Nationalities and People's Regional Government
FGD	Focus Group Discussion
IPA	Interpretive Phenomenological Analysis
ICPD	International Conference on Population and Development

A. Profile of study participants

A. 1 FGD

Site 1

See **Tables A1–A9**.

S. No.	Age	Education	# of children	Year of contraceptive use
1	35	9	4	5
2	25	10	4	10
3	30	5	8	10
4	32	1	03	7
5	30	6	05	12
6	25	4	4	6
7	35	7	7	10
8	25	—	5	3
9	27	10+3	2	6
10	32	2	7	8
11	30	9	7	6
Mean	**29.64**		**5.1**	**7.54**

Table A1.
Profile extracted from the FGD participants' transcription document of the Waycho site.

Site 2

S. No.	Age	Education	# of children	Year of contraceptive use
1	25	7	5	4
2	30	—	8	7
3	25	6	3	4
4	25	—	4	3
5	34	8	4	3
6	30	—	8	2
7	40	6	8	6
8	20	10 completed	1	2
9	40	4	7	7
10	25	3	2	4
Mean	**29.4**	**4.4**	5	**4.2**

Table A2.
Profile of the participants extracted from the FGD participants' transcription document of the Ganie site.

Site 3

S. No.	Age	Education	# of children	Year of contraceptive use
1	28	—	4	3.5
2	27	—	5	7
3	23	10 completed	1	2.5
4	25	—	7	4
5	30	—	4	10
6	30	—	6	8
7	25	—	4	8
8	20	4	3	4
9	30	—	6	6
Mean	26.44		4.44	5.88

Table A3.
Profile of the participants extracted from the FGD participants' transcription document of the Degara site.

Site 4

S. No.	Age	Education	# of children	Year of contraceptive use
1	28	—	6	3
2	27	—	5	7
3	30	—	4	3
4	35	—	3	1
5	30	—	6	4
6	30	—	8	5
7	25	—	5	2
8	30	3	5	2
Mean	29.4		5.25	3.34

Table A4.
Profile of the participants extracted from the FGD participants' transcription document of the Korangoge site.

DOI: http://dx.doi.org/10.5772/intechopen.111694

Site 5

S. No.	Age	Education	# of children	Year of contraceptive use
1	25	5	5	8
2	22	8	3	4
3	20	4	4	3
4	20	9	2	2
5	25	6	5	5
6	26	6	5	9
7	20	4	2	3
Mean	22.57	6	3.7	4.86

Table A5.
Profile of the participants extracted from the FGD participants' transcription document of the Dilarife site.

Site 6

S. No	Age	Education	# of children ever born	Period of contraceptive use	Remark
1	25	5	2	5 years	
2	25	4	5	7	
3	22	7	1	1 and half	
4	35	3	7	5 and 3/12	
5	30	—	4	4	
6	30	—	6	3	
7	22	10 completed	1	2	
Mean	**27**	**4.14**	**3.7**	**4**	

Table A6.
Profile of the participants extracted from the FGD participants' transcription document of the Konsore Fullasa site.

Site 7

S. No	Age	Education	# of children ever born	Period of contraceptive use	Remark
1	36	8	10	5 years	
2	28	5	3	1	
3	30	2	6	8	
4	30	5	4	1	
5	34	2	4	3.5	
6	32	-	4	3.5	
7	35	7	5	11	
8	30	-	2	4	
9	25	3	3	5	
10	30	7	5	9	
Mean	**31**	**3.9**	**4.6**	**5**	

Table A7.
Profile of the participants extracted from the FGD participants' transcription document of the Gassara Kuwie site.

Site 8

S. No	Age	Education	# of children ever born	Period of contraceptive use	Remark
1	25	7	2	3 years	
2	30	1	4	8	
3	35	—	5	9 and half	
4	30	—	5	7	
5	25	—	3	3	
6	38	5	4	6	
7	30	—	5	8	
8	30	—	4	13	
Mean	**30.38**	**1.63**	**4**	**7.2**	

Table A8.
Profile of the participants extracted from the FGD participants' transcription document of the Wotara Gendo site.

Site 9

S. No	Age	Education	# of children ever born	Period of contraceptive use	Remark
1	36	8	10	5 years	
2	30	5	3	1	
3	35	2	6	8	
4	30	5	4	1	
5	30	-	4	3.5	
6	35	-	4	3.5	
7	35	7	5	11	
8	30	-	2	4	
9	20	3	3	5	
10	30	7	5	9	
11	35	5	4	5	
12	35	6	7	6	
Mean	31.75	4	4.75	5.16	

Table A9.
Profile of the participants extracted from the FGD participants' transcription document of the Basha site.

A. 2 Profile of key informants

See **Table A10**.

S. no.	Age	Sex	Education	Profession	Service YR	Position
1	30	M	BSc	Health Officer	12	District Head
2	28	M	BSc	Health Officer	2	Deputy Head, district
3	27	M	BSc	Nurse	4	District Head
4	34	M	BSc	Health Officer	13	RH coordinator, District
5	29	M	BSc	Family science	7	RH coordinator, District
6	51	M	BSc	Health Officer	31	RH coordinator, HC
7	29	F	Diploma	Clinical Nurse	4	RH coordinator, HC
8	26	F	10 + 1	Health Extension W	7	Service provide
9	30	F	10 + 1	Health Extension W	8	Service provide
10	22	F	10 + 1	Health Extension W	7	Service provide
11	25	F	10 + 1	Health Extension W	7	Service provide
12	44	M	BSc	Nurse	27	RH coordinator, HC
13	25	F	Diploma	Midwife	5	RH coordinator, HC
14	23	F	10 + 1	Health Extension W	8	Service provide
15	28	M	MD + MPH	Physician	7	Director for RH, Federal Minister of Health
16	38	M	MPH	Public health	18	Deputy Head Regional Health Bureau
17	25	F	10 + 1	Health Extension W	7	Service provide
18	23	F	10 + 1	Health Extension W	7	Service provide

N.B. The Key informants composed of service providers at community and health institution levels, health service managers at district, regional and federal levels indicating the hierarchy.

Table A10.
Key informant profile extracted from the transcription of the informants' document from the study sites such as health institutions (health post and health center) and the health services administrative offices.

B. Data analysis flow diagram adapted from IPAThe qualitative data analysis steps adapted from IPA (Smith et al., 2009, pp. 82–100) and customized to fit my study taking the following steps as indicated below in flow diagram (Figure B1).

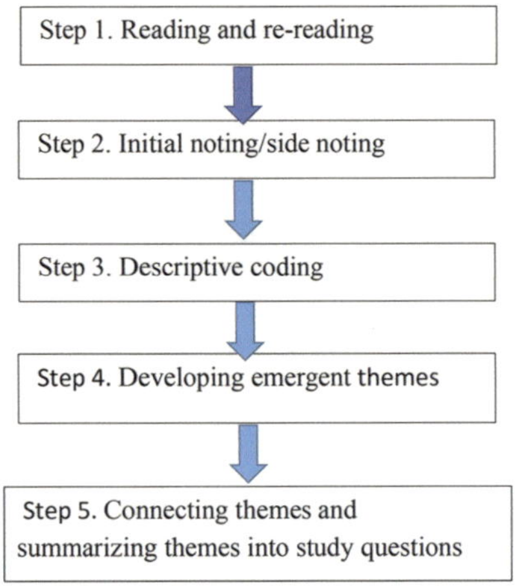

Figure B1.
It can be cited as Fig. B1. Flow diagram of data analysis adapted from the Interpretive Phenomenological Analysis (IPA).

C. A flow diagram indicating steps in translation

This study involved several participants in the overall processes with various languages background. In order to establish a common understanding and create

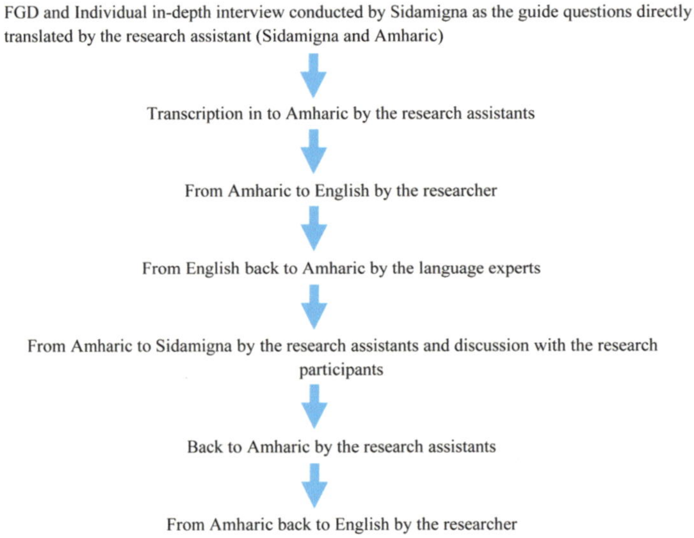

Figure C1.
This can be cited as a flow diagram developed to indicate a translation of transcription from the local language to the working language in the stepwise (developed by the researcher).

closeness in the process of the research, use of language translation from one to another has been a necessary condition. Accordingly, the following steps in translation has been taken until the final text took its recent shape (**Figure C1**).

Author details

Abraham Alano[1*] and Lori Hanson[2]

1 SNNPR Policy Research Institute, Hawassa University, College of Medicine and Health Sciences, School of Public Health, SNNPR, Hawassa, Ethiopia

2 Department of Community Health and Epidemiology, College of Medicine, University of Saskatchewan, Saskatoon, Canada

*Address all correspondence to: alanoabraham@yahoo.com

References

[1] Bongaarts J, Sinding SW. A response to family planning programs. International Perspectives on Sexual and Reproductive Health. 2009;**35**(1):39-44

[2] Cleland J. Contraception in historical and global perspectives. Best Practice and Research Clinical Obstetrics and Gynaecology. 2008;**23**:165-176

[3] Seltzer JR. The origin and evolution family planning programms in developing countries. RAND. 2002

[4] McLaren A. A History of Contraception from Antiquity to the Present Day. Oxford: Blackwell; 1990

[5] Harkavy O, Roy K. Emergence of the Indian family planning program. In: Robinson WC, Ross JA, editors. The Global Family Planning Revolution: Three Decades of Population Policies and Programs. Washington DC: The World Bank; 2007

[6] Westoff CF, Cross A. The Stall in the Fertility Transition in Kenya. Calverton: ORC Macro, Demographic and Health Surveys Analytic Studies; 2006

[7] Haggerty J, Burge F, Lévesque JF, Gass D, Pineault R, Beaulieu MD, et al. Operational definitions of attributes of primary health care: Consensus among Canadian Experts. Annals of Family Medicine. 2007;**5**:336-344

[8] Walraven G. The 2018 Astana declaration on primary health care, is it useful?. Journal of Global Health. 2019;**9**(1)

[9] WHO & UNICEF. Primary Health Care Report of the International Conference on Primary Health Care. Alma-Ata: USSR; 6-12 Sept 1978

[10] Perry HP, Zulliger R, Rogers MM. Community health workers in low-, middle-, and high-income countries: An overview of their history, recent evolution, and current effectiveness. Annual Review of Public Health. 2014;**35**:399-421

[11] Ministry of Finance and Economic Development (MOFED). Ethiopia: Building on Progress: Plan for Accelerated and Sustained Development to End Poverty (2005/6-2009/10) (PASDEP). Addis Ababa; 2005

[12] Transitional Government of Ethiopia [TGE]. Health Policy of the Transitional Government of Ethiopia. Ethiopia: Addis Ababa; 1993

[13] Workie NW, Ramana GN. The Health Extension Program in Ethiopia. UNICO Studies series 10. Washington DC: The World bank; 2013

[14] Center for Health and Gender Equity. Women's Sexual and Reproductive Health and Rights in Ethiopia: The Role of the National Government and U.S. Foreign Assistance. Washington, DC: Center for Health and Gender Equity; 2010

[15] Teklehaimanot HD, Teklehaimanot A. Human resource development for a community based health extension program: A case study of Ethiopia. BMC. Human Resource for Health. 2013;**11**(39):1-12. Available from: http://www.human-resource-health.com/content/11/1/39

[16] Health system 20/20-USAID (2012). Health Extension Program: An Innovative Solution to Public Health Challenges of Ethiopia. A Case Study. Ethiopia: Addis Ababa; 2012

[17] FMOH. National Reproductive Health Strategy (2006-2015). Ethiopi: Addis Ababa; 2006

[18] FMOH. Health Sector Development Plan IV, 2010/11-2014/15. Ethiopia: Addis Ababa; 2010

[19] United States Aid for International Development (USAID). Promoting Urban Health and Launch of the Strengthening Ethiopia's Urban Health Extension Program (SEUHP). Ethiopia: Addis Ababa; 2014

[20] Central Statistical Authority of Ethiopia (CSA, E). Population and Housing Census. Addis Ababa: CS; 2008

[21] Sidama Zone Health Department. Sidama Zonal Health Profile. unpublished; 2012

[22] Morse JM, Niehaus L. Combining qualitative and quantitative methods for mixed method designs. In: Munhall PL, editor. Nursing Research: A Qualitative Perespectives. 5th ed. Jones & Bartelet Learning: Miami, Florida; 2012. pp. 571-584

[23] Flood A. Understanding phenomenology. Nursing Research. 2010;**17**(2):7-15

[24] Munhall PL. Nursing Research. A Qualitative Perspective. Fifth ed. Miam, Filorida: Jones & Bartlet Learning; 2012

[25] Denzin NK, Lincoln YS. Introduction: The discipline and practice of qualitative research. In: Denzin NK, Lincoln YS, editors. Handbook of Qualitative Research. 2nd ed. Thousand Oaks, CA: Sage; 2000. pp. 1-29

[26] Patton MQ. Qualitative Research and Evaluation Methods. 3rd ed. Thousand Oaks, CA: Sage; 2002

[27] vanManen M. Researching Lived Experience: Human Science for an Action Sensitive Pedagogy. 2nd ed. London, Ontario, Canada: Althouse Press; 1997

[28] Krueger RA, Casey MA. Focus Groups: A Practical Guide for Applied Research (4thEd.). Thousand Oaks, CA: Sage Publications; 2009

[29] Lopez KA, Willis DG. Descriptive versus interpretive phenomenology: Their contributions to nursing knowledge. Qualitative Health Research. 2004;**14**(5):726-735. DOI: 10.1177/1049732304263638

[30] Wojnar DM, Swanson KM. Phenomenology: An exploration. Journal of Holistic Nursing. 2007;**25**(3):172-180

[31] Curtin M, Fossey E. Appraising the trustworthiness of qualitative studies: Guidelines for occupational therapists. Australian Occupational Therapy Journal. 2007;**54**(2):88-94

[32] Rolfe G. Validity, trustworthiness and rigour: Quality and the idea of qualitative research. Journal of Advanced Nursing. 2006;**53**(3):304-310

[33] Morrow SL. Quality and trustworthiness in qualitative research in counseling psychology. Journal of Counseling Psychology. 2005;**52**(2):250-260

[34] Karim AM, Bieze B, Chimnani J. Measuring Family Planning Logistics System Performance in Developing Countries: Working Paper. Arlington, VA: USAID | DELIVER PROJECT, Task Order 1; 2008. Available from: http://deliver.jsi.com/dlvr_content/resources/allpubs/policypapers/MeasFPLogiSyst_WP.pdf

[35] MSH (Management Services for Health). Cultural Competent Organizations. 2011. Available from:

http://erc.msh.org/mainpage.cfm?file=9.1.htm&module=provider&language=English. [Accessed: March 8, 2011]

[36] Prata N, Gessessew A, Cartwright A, Fraser A. Provision of injectable contraceptives in Ethiopia through community based reproductive health agents. In: Bulletin of World Health Organization. Vol. 89. Ethiopia: Progress, Achievements and Challenges. Addis Ababa, World Health Organization; 2011. pp. 556-564

[37] Central Statistical Authority (CSA) & ORC Macro. Ethiopia Demographic and Health Survey. Addis Abab: CSA; 2011

[38] Central Statistical Authority of Ethiopia (CSA) & ORC Macro. Ethiopia Demographic and Health Survey Report 2005. Addis Ababa and Calverton: Central Statistical Authority and ORC Macro; 2006

[39] Chaya N. Poor access to health services: Ways Ethiopia overcoming it. Research Commentary. 2007;**2**(2):1-6

[40] Hoke T, Brune A, Kruger K, Dreisbach C, Akol A, Stanback J. community- based distribution of injectable contraceptives: Introduction strategies in four sub-Saharan African countries. International Perspectives on Sexual and Reproductive Health. 2012;**38**(4):214-219

[41] Obrist B, Iteba N, Lengeler C, Makemba A, Mshana C, et al. Access to health care in contexts of livelihood insecurity: A framework for analysis and action. PLoS Medicine. 2007;**4**(10):e308

[42] Provincial Health Service Authority. Towards Reducing Health Inequalities. A Health Systems Approach to Chronic Diseases Prevention. A discussion paper. Vancouver, BC: Population and Public Health; 2011

[43] World Health Organization (WHO). Optimizing Health Worker Roles to Improve Access to Key Maternal and Newborn Health Interventions through Task Shifting. Geneva: WHO Department of Reproductive Health and Research; 2012. Available from: http://apps.who.int/iris/bitstream/10665/77764/1/9789241504843_eng.pdf www.,ccsenet.org/gihs

[44] Wickstrom J, Yanulis J, van Lith L, Jones B. Mobile outreach services for family planning: A descriptive inquiry in Malawi, Nepal, and Tanzanai. The RESPOND Project Study Series. 2013;**13**

[45] Gulzar J, Ali M, Kuroiwa C. A social marketing approach to quality improvement in family planning services: A case study from Rawalindi, Pakistan. Biosciences Trends. 2008;**2**(1):15-21

[46] Hardee K, Kumar J, Newman K, Bakamjian L, Harris S, Rodirguez M, et al. Voluntary, human right-based family planning: A conceptual framework. Studies in Family Planning. 2014;**45**(1):1-18